Contemporary Perspectives on Social Work in Acquired Brain Injury

T0174627

Contemporary Perspectives is the first book to address social work practice in the field of brain injury (BI). Contributions are written by social work authors from around the world, and highlight the diversity of social work practice and theory within this field. Chapters range from practice spanning interventions with families caring for a child with BI; interventions to assist the adjustment of families facing the challenge of supporting an adult relative with BI during the inpatient rehabilitation or post-acute community phase; work with parents with BI who are caring for children deemed to be at risk; and a literature review outlining the impact of a BI on siblings. Other chapters detail a program for self-advocacy; investigate the impact of violence-related BI; evaluate a peer-support program for people with BI; report on the role of support people in facilitating return to work after BI; and examine the role of social work within the interdisciplinary rehabilitation team.

The volume highlights the valuable role social work makes to the field of BI and contributes to the knowledge base informing evidence-informed practice within this field.

This book was originally published as a special issue of the *Journal of Social Work in Disability & Rehabilitation*.

Grahame K. Simpson is an Associate Professor at the Ingham Institute of Applied Medical Research, Sydney, Australia, where he leads the Brain Injury Rehabilitation Research Group. He has over 30 years practice and research experience in brain injury rehabilitation and is founding co-convenor of the International Network of Social Workers in Acquired Brain Injury.

Francis Yuen is a Social Work Professor at California State University, Sacramento, USA. He has published widely and served as the editor for the *Journal of Social Work in Disability & Rehabilitation* since 2003. He has been a principal investigator, evaluator, and trainer for national and local service organizations.

Contemporary Perspectives on Social Work in Acquired Brain Injury

Edited by
Grahame K. Simpson and Francis Yuen

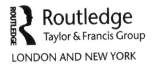

Routledge
Taylor & Francis Group

LONDON AND NEW YORK

First published 2018 by Routledge

2 Park Square, Milton Park, Abingdon, Oxfordshire OX14 4RN
52 Vanderbilt Avenue, New York, NY 10017

Routledge is an imprint of the Taylor & Francis Group, an informa business

First issued in paperback 2019

British Library Cataloguing in Publication Data
A catalogue record for this book is available from the British Library

ISBN 13: 978-1-138-55974-5 (hbk)
ISBN 13: 978-0-367-89214-2 (pbk)

Typeset in Minion Pro
by RefineCatch Limited, Bungay, Suffolk

Publisher's Note
The publisher accepts responsibility for any inconsistencies that may have
arisen during the conversion of this book from journal articles to book chapters,
namely the possible inclusion of journal terminology.

Disclaimer
Every effort has been made to contact copyright holders for their permission to
reprint material in this book. The publishers would be grateful to hear from any
copyright holder who is not here acknowledged and will undertake to rectify
any errors or omissions in future editions of this book.

Contents

CONTENTS

Citation Information

The chapters in this book were originally published in the *Journal of Social Work in Disability & Rehabilitation*, volume 15, issue 3–4 (2016). When citing this material, please use the original page numbering for each article, as follows:

Introduction
Contemporary Perspectives on Social Work in Acquired Brain Injury: An Introduction
Grahame Simpson and Francis Yuen
Journal of Social Work in Disability & Rehabilitation, volume 15, issue 3–4 (2016),
pp. 169–178

Chapter 1
Family Forward: Promoting Family Adaptation Following Pediatric Acquired Brain Injury
Lyndal Hickey, Vicki Anderson, and Brigid Jordan
Journal of Social Work in Disability & Rehabilitation, volume 15, issue 3–4 (2016),
pp. 179–200

Chapter 2
Self-Advocacy for Independent Life: A Program for Personal Self Advocacy after Brain Injury
Lenore A. Hawley
Journal of Social Work in Disability & Rehabilitation, volume 15, issue 3–4 (2016),
pp. 201–212

Chapter 3
Describing an Early Social Work Intervention Program for Families after Severe Traumatic Brain Injury
Grahame Simpson, Daniella Pfeiffer, Shay Keogh, and Brigitte Lane
Journal of Social Work in Disability & Rehabilitation, volume 15, issue 3–4 (2016),
pp. 213–233

Chapter 4
Acquired Brain Injury, Parenting, Social Work, and Rehabilitation: Supporting Parents to Support Their Children
Mark Holloway and Lauren Tyrrell
Journal of Social Work in Disability & Rehabilitation, volume 15, issue 3–4 (2016),
pp. 234–259

Chapter 5

Mindful Connections: The Role of a Peer Support Group on the Psychosocial Adjustment for Adults Recovering From Brain Injury
Melissa Cutler, Michelle L. A. Nelson, Maya Nikoloski, and Kerry Kuluski
Journal of Social Work in Disability & Rehabilitation, volume 15, issue 3–4 (2016), pp. 260–284

Chapter 6

Holding Resilience in Trust: Working Systemically With Families Following an Acquired Brain Injury
Franca Butera-Prinzi, Nella Charles, and Karen Story
Journal of Social Work in Disability & Rehabilitation, volume 15, issue 3–4 (2016), pp. 285–304

Chapter 7

Brain Injury as the Result of Violence: A Systematic Scoping Review
Annerley Bates, Sarah Matthews, Grahame Simpson, and Lyndel Bates
Journal of Social Work in Disability & Rehabilitation, volume 15, issue 3–4 (2016), pp. 305–331

Chapter 8

A Clarion Call for Social Work Attention: Brothers and Sisters of Persons With Acquired Brain Injury in the United States
Charles Edmund Degeneffe
Journal of Social Work in Disability & Rehabilitation, volume 15, issue 3–4 (2016), pp. 332–350

Chapter 9

Support Persons' Perceptions of Giving Vocational Rehabilitation Support to Clients With Acquired Brain Injury in Sweden
Marie Matérne, Lars-Olov Lundqvist, and Thomas Strandberg
Journal of Social Work in Disability & Rehabilitation, volume 15, issue 3–4 (2016), pp. 351–369

Chapter 10

Social Workers' Perceived Role Clarity as Members of an Interdisciplinary Team in Brain Injury Settings
Martha Vungkhanching and Kareen N. Tonsing
Journal of Social Work in Disability & Rehabilitation, volume 15, issue 3–4 (2016), pp. 370–384

For any permission-related enquiries please visit:
http://www.tandfonline.com/page/help/permissions

Notes on Contributors

Vicki Anderson is a Pediatric Neuropsychologist; Director of Psychology at the Royal Children's Hospital; and Director, Clinical Sciences Research, Murdoch Children's Research Institute, Australia.

Annerley Bates, PhD, is a Senior Social Worker with the Brain Injury Rehabilitation Service at the Princess Alexandra Hospital, Queensland, Australia.

Lyndel Bates is a Lecturer in the School of Criminology and Criminal Justice and a member of the Griffith Criminology Institute at Griffith University, Australia.

Franca Butera-Prinzi is a Social Worker and Family Therapist with 30 years of experience. She is currently the Team Leader of the Acquired Brain Injury team at The Bouverie Centre, Australia, and Acting Clinical Program Manager.

Nella Charles is a Family Therapist and Psychologist at The Bouverie Centre, Australia, where she is employed on a part-time basis as a clinician and teacher in family therapy.

Melissa Cutler is a Clinical Social Worker who has specialized in the field of neurorehabilitation and mental health for 15 years. She works within the Ambulatory Care Program at Sinai Health System–Bridgepoint Site in Toronto, Canada.

Charles Edmund Degeneffe is a Professor of Rehabilitation Counseling at San Diego State University (SDSU), USA. He is the Coordinator of the SDSU Masters in Rehabilitation Counseling Program and SDSU Certificate Program in Cognitive Disabilities.

Lenore A. Hawley is a licensed Clinical Social Worker and certified brain injury specialist trainer. She is the Brain Injury Education and Resource Counselor at Craig Hospital in Englewood, USA, where she also serves as a research clinician and GIST group therapist. She is a member of the Executive Committee of the International Network for Social Workers in Acquired Brain Injury.

Lyndal Hickey is a Senior Rehabilitation Social Worker at the Royal Children's Hospital, Melbourne, Australia. She is a member of the International Network of Social Workers in Acquired Brain Injury and Victorian Subacute Childhood Stroke Advisory Committee.

Mark Holloway is a UK qualified and registered Social Worker with 25 years of experience working with people with an acquired brain injury. He is an advanced member of the British Association of Brain Injury Case Managers.

Brigid Jordan is an Associate Professor of Pediatric Social Work at the Royal Children's Hospital, Melbourne and the Department of Pediatrics at the University of Melbourne, Australia, and heads the Social and Mental Health Research Group at the Murdoch Children's Research Institute, Australia.

Shay Keogh is currently employed as a Social Worker with Queensland Health working in Caboolture and Kilcoy hospitals, Australia. She has worked for the past 17 years in a range of health-related social work fields including brain injury rehabilitation and aged care.

Kerry Kuluski is a scientist at the Lunenfeld-Tanenbaum Research Institute, Sinai Health System, Canada, and Assistant Professor at the Institute of Health Policy, Management, and Evaluation, Dalla Lana School of Public Health, University of Toronto, Canada.

Brigitte Lane received her Doctorate of Clinical Psychology from the University of Sydney, Australia. She has contributed to research in brain injury rehabilitation whilst at Liverpool Brain Injury Rehabilitation Unit, and more recently in eating disorders. She has worked in community and hospital settings for general mental health in New Zealand and Sydney.

Lars-Olov Lundqvist is an Associate Professor in Psychology and Research Leader at the University Health Care Research Center, Örebro University, Sweden, and former Head of the Centre for Rehabilitation Research, Region Örebro County. He has a broad background in psychology, with specific expertise in epidemiological, psychometric, and experimental research in affective neuroscience.

Marie Matérne is a Social Worker. She is working part-time as a business developer for Habiliation and assistive technology in Region Örebro County, Sweden, and part-time as a PhD candidate in Disability Research, her project is about return to work after acquired brain injury. She is a member of the Executive Committee of the International Network of Social Workers in Acquired Brain Injury.

Sarah Matthews received her Bachelors of Psychological Science from Griffith University, Brisbane, Australia. She has been involved in the Assault and Brain Injuries project since 2014, which aims to investigate assault-related traumatic brain injury and its impact on caregivers. She also has research assistance experience on a diverse range of projects.

Michelle L. A. Nelson is a Research Scientist at the Bridgepoint Collaboratory, Lunenfeld-Tanenbaum Research Institute, Canada. She has academic appointments in the Daphne Cockwell School of Nursing at Ryerson University, Canada, and the Dalla Lana School of Public Health, Division of Clinical Public Health, at the University of Toronto, Canada.

Maya Nikoloski currently works as the Manager of Professional Practice Nursing at Bridgepoint Hospital, Sinai Health System, Canada. She is engaged in professional development and academia through her Adjunct Lecturer appointment with the Lawrence S. Bloomberg Faculty of Nursing, University of Toronto, Canada.

Daniella Pfeiffer has 10 years of clinical experience as a Social Worker specializing in brain injury rehabilitation. She is a Senior Project Officer delivering education and training to allied health professionals across NSW Health, Australia.

Grahame K. Simpson is an Associate Professor at the Ingham Institute of Applied Medical Research, Sydney, Australia, where he leads the Brain Injury Rehabilitation Research Group. He has over 30 years practice and research experience in brain injury rehabilitation and is founding co-convenor of the International Network of Social Workers in Acquired Brain Injury.

Karen Story is a Social Worker, Child and Adolescent Psychotherapist, and Family Therapist. She has extensive experience working with individuals and families as a Senior Psychotherapist and Clinical Mental Health Social Worker at Austin CAMHS and in private practice. She is currently a Family Therapist on the Acquired Brain Injury team.

Thomas Strandberg is an Associate Professor in Caring Sciences and Disability Research at Örebro University, Sweden, and the Swedish Institute for Disability Research. He is a member of the board of the Nordic Network on Disability Research.

Kareen N. Tonsing is an Assistant Professor of Social Work at Oakland University, USA. She was awarded her PhD from The University of Hong Kong. Her research interests include acculturation, psychological adaptation, children and family welfare, mental health, and domestic violence. She is a licensed Social Worker and has worked with diverse client populations in Hong Kong.

Lauren Tyrrell has been the clinical lead Social Worker with the Trauma Team at the McKellar Community Rehabilitation Centre in Geelong, Australia, since 2010. She is currently completing a master's in Family Therapy, and is a member of the Australian Association of Social Workers.

Martha Vungkhanching is Professor and Chair in the Department of Social Work Education at California State University, Fresno, USA. She has extensive practice experience in substance abuse treatment and rehabilitation. Her research interests include alcohol and substance abuse, traumatic brain injury, oncology social work, health and mental health, and international social work practice.

Francis Yuen is a Social Work Professor at California State University, Sacramento, USA. He has published widely and served as the editor for the *Journal of Social Work in Disability & Rehabilitation* since 2003. He has been a principal investigator, evaluator, and trainer for national and local service organizations.

Contemporary Perspectives on Social Work in Acquired Brain Injury: An Introduction

Grahame Simpson and Francis Yuen

ABSTRACT

This special issue of the Journal of Social Work in Disability and Rehabilitation, "Contemporary Perspectives on Social Work in Acquired Brain Injury," has been initiated and coordinated by the International Network of Social Workers in Acquired Brain Injury (INSWABI). In introducing the issue, some space is allocated for providing definitions of traumatic brain injury (TBI) and acquired brain injury (ABI), outlining the epidemiology and global costs, and detailing the impairments and psycho-social impacts for both the person sustaining the injury and his or her family. Finally, an outline of the articles contributing to this special issue are detailed, followed by a brief discussion about the role of the INSWABI network in promoting best practice in social work within this specialty area.

Acquired brain injury (ABI) is a major global health issue. It is prevalent across both the developed and developing world. It can have devastating effects on the individual and their families. It also has major societal costs including premature mortality; significant levels of acute health service use and high morbidity amongst those who survive; lost productivity; and the need for longer term formal and informal care. Social workers encounter people with ABI and their families in a variety of settings along the continuum of care from emergency departments and acute inpatient medical/sub-acute rehabilitation wards through to outpatient services and longer term community rehabilitation and disability support services. Despite the growth in numbers of people living with ABI encountered by social workers, there has been very little published work to guide social workers in their practice within this field. The first part of this chapter provides a brief introduction to the field, starting with one particular sub-type, traumatic brain injury (TBI), and then moving outwards to address other forms of ABI. The second half of the chapter provides an outline of the remainder of the book and some background about the International Network of Social Workers in ABI, the e-network behind this initiative.

In an international consensus-based definition, traumatic brain injury (TBI) has been characterized as "an alteration in brain function, or other evidence of brain pathology, caused by an external force" (Menon, Schwab, Wright, & Maas, 2010, p. 1638). In most cases, this alteration in brain function involves some change to the level of consciousness or the presence of posttraumatic amnesia (PTA). PTA is "a state of generalized cognitive disturbance characterized by confusion, disorientation, retrograde amnesia, inability to store new memories, and sometimes agitation and delusions" (Ponsford, Janzen, et al., 2014, p. 307) on behalf of the INCOG Expert Panel.

Causes of injury include falls, assaults, road accidents, gunshots, sporting injuries, blast injuries, or natural disasters. The types of TBI caused by such events include closed head injuries (e.g., when the brain damage is caused by acceleration and deceleration or rotational forces applied to the brain, causing primary injuries such as hemorrhages, hematomas, or diffuse axonal injury), penetrating injuries (e.g., when an object, such as a bullet, pierces the skull and directly inflicts damage on underlying brain tissue), blast injuries (most commonly arising in conflict zones from exposure to pressure waves generated by the detonation of improvised explosive devices; Rona et al., 2012), or finally and less frequently, crush injuries (e.g., compression of the skull, usually arising from being caught between two hard surfaces, as might occur from being caught in a building that has collapsed during an earthquake; Lateef, 2011).

The three most common approaches to classifying severity of TBI include two measures of initial injury severity and one measure of longer term outcome. The Glasgow Coma Scale categorizes initial injury severity as mild, moderate, or severe (Teasdale, 1995; Teasdale & Jennett, 1974). The other common approach to assessing initial injury severity is the measurement of duration of PTA, which encompasses mild (< 60 min), moderate (1–24 hr), and various gradations of severe including severe (1–7 days), very severe (1–4 weeks) and extremely severe (greater than 4 weeks; Jennett & Teasdale, 1981; Russell & Smith, 1961; Teasdale, 1995). Finally, the Glasgow Outcome Scale (Jennett, Snoek, Bond, & Brooks, 1981) categorizes longer term outcomes in five categories, namely dead, persistent vegetative state, severe disability, moderate disability, and good recovery.

TBI is one form of acquired brain injury (ABI). ABI can be defined as "damage to the brain which occurs after birth" (Australian Institute of Health and Welfare, 2007, p. 1). In addition to traumatic causes, ABI comprises other nonprogressive conditions including stroke (including cerebral aneurysms), infections (e.g., encephalitis or meningitis), toxins (e.g., alcohol in alcohol-related brain damage), and anoxia or hypoxia (i.e., when the oxygen flow to the brain is reduced or ceases, as can occur in a near drowning, hanging, or drug overdose). There is less consensus about whether progressive conditions (e.g., brain tumor, dementia, multiple sclerosis) also fall under the umbrella of ABI, or are otherwise classed (e.g., as progressive or neurodegenerative disorders).

The articles in this special issue range from studies with exclusive samples of people with TBI (or the carers and relatives of people with TBI), through to work addressing people with brain injury arising from the broader range of etiologies encompassed within ABI. In terms of age range, the studies focus on children, adolescents, or adults of working age, but not the elderly, reflecting the main focus of the International Network of Social Workers in Acquired Brain Injury (INSWABI; i.e., people who acquired their brain injury between the ages of 0–65 years). Overall, the predominant focus of the studies is on TBI and so the following paragraphs address this form of ABI.

A meta-analysis of epidemiological studies across Europe found an incidence rate of 262 per 100,000 people with TBI hospitalized each year, spanning all categories of injury severity (Peeters et al., 2015). In the United States, it is estimated that 1.4 million TBIs occur every year (Langlois, Rutland-Brown, & Wald, 2006). TBI has a bimodal distribution, with injuries most common among people under the age of 25 or over the age of 75 (Peeters et al., 2015). In all studies, there is a higher male-to-female ratio, ranging from a low of 1.2:1.0 up to the highest ratio of 4.6:1.0 (Peeters et al., 2015). In most epidemiological studies, about 80% of injuries are mild, with smaller proportions of moderate and severe injuries (Langlois et al., 2006; Peeters et al., 2015; Tate, McDonald, & Lulham, 1998). The most common cause of injury varies with the degree of severity. Overall, the most common cause of injury is falls (Langlois et al., 2006; Tate et al., 1998). However, for the subgroup with severe injuries, road accidents are still the most common cause (Tate et al., 1998).

Estimates of the prevalence vary widely, with population studies and meta-analyses of epidemiological studies finding that between 5% and 12% of the population across different Western countries self-report having a TBI (Anstey et al., 2004; Frost, Farrer, Primosch, & Hedges, 2013). The estimated annual health care costs associated with all TBI (mild, moderate, and severe) in the United States are US$60 billion (Finkelstein, Corso, & Miller, 2006); in Australia, the estimated cost for all TBI is AU$8.6 billion (Access Economics, 2009). Therefore, reducing the mortality and morbidity associated with TBI is an important health and social priority.

Impairments of TBI can be grouped into motor/sensory, cognitive, communication, and behavioral domains. The great majority of people make a good physical recovery after TBI (in contrast to stroke, which has much higher rates of physical disability), with few requiring mobility aids (Ponsford, Downing, et al., 2014). However, neurological impairments such as loss of sense of taste, vision impairments, headaches, and problems with balance are still observed up to 10 years postinjury (Ponsford, Downing, et al., 2014).

Only a minority of people have global cognitive impairments post-TBI. In the great majority of cases, people have a mix of preserved cognitive abilities intermingled with areas of difficulty. The cognitive impairments that are most commonly encountered include slower speed of information processing, attentional difficulties, problems with memory, and impairments in executive function (Ponsford, Sloan, & Snow, 2013). Executive function includes higher order cognitive processing associated with planning, organizing, goal setting, problem solving, self-awareness, and monitoring of behavior (Ponsford et al., 2013). Cognitive communication changes (i.e., communication changes resulting from primary cognitive impairments) can span listening, speaking, reading, writing, conversation, and social interaction (College of Audiologists and Speech-Language Pathologists of Ontario, 2002). Finally, behavioral changes can include impulsivity, self-centeredness, and increased anger or aggression, or alternatively, disinhibition, apathy, and problems with initiation (Ponsford et al., 2013; Sabaz et al., 2014).

Despite these challenges, most adults with severe TBI will regain their independence in everyday living. There are far greater problems in gaining or regaining meaningful occupation (e.g., only 30–40% of people with severe TBI will return to paid employment postinjury; Tate, Simpson, & McRae, 2015). Similarly, maintaining existing relationships, such as marriages (Wood & Yurdakul, 1997) or friendships (Rowlands, 2000), or developing new relationships is not easy. Finally, the social impact of TBI can include increased risk of substance abuse (Bogner & Corrigan, 2013), mental health problems (Gould, Ponsford, Johnston, & Schönberger, 2011; Tsaousides, Ashman, & Gordon, 2013), homelessness (Oddy, Moir, Fortescue, & Chadwick, 2012), social isolation (Rowlands, 2000), incarceration (Williams et al., 2010), unemployment (Tyerman, 2012), and suicide (Simpson & Tate, 2007).

Families play an important role after TBI, and often become the key support for the person with TBI. Families enhance outcomes (Barclay, 2013; Sander et al., 2003). However, families can face many challenges in providing support to their relatives. In particular, the cognitive and behavioral changes associated with TBI are more challenging for carers to deal with than the physical sequelae (Anderson et al., 2009). Furthermore, many caregivers report elevated levels of depression, anxiety, and stress in comparison to the general population, with rates ranging between 20% and 40% (Anderson, Simpson, & Morey, 2013; Anderson et al., 2009; Kruetzer et al., 2009). Changes in the dynamics of family functioning are also reported, including reduced affective involvement, communication, general functioning, and role change (Anderson et al., 2013; Anderson et al., 2009; Kruetzer et al., 2009). Despite the challenges, many families show surprising levels of resilience and adaptive coping abilities (Perlesz, Kinsella, & Crowe, 1999; Simpson & Jones, 2013)

Carlton and Stephenson (1990) commented that given the broad biopsychosocial impact of TBI, it was surprising that social workers had not published more on the subject. The articles in this special issue represent a step in this direction. The contributions highlight several fronts on which social workers, in collaboration with their colleagues from other disciplines, are conducting cutting-edge research in the field of TBI and ABI.

Encouragingly, 6 of the 10 articles focus on practice delivery, including two intervention study protocols, outlining manualized programs currently being evaluated by means of randomized controlled trials: the Family Forward program, which aims to build resilient adaptation among families with children who have sustained an ABI (Hickey, Anderson, & Jordan) and the Self-Advocacy for Independent Life (SAIL) program, providing training in self-advocacy skills for people with ABI and their family members (Hawley). Furthermore, four other studies describe or evaluate existing practice; namely early intervention social work services provided to families in an inpatient brain injury rehabilitation setting (Simpson, Pfeiffer, Keogh, & Lane); work with parents with ABI who are caring for children deemed to be at risk (Holloway & Tyrrell); a postacute, group-based, psychosocial peer support program for adults with ABI under the age of 55 (Cutler, Nelson, Nikoloski, & Kuluski); and a study looking critically at the construct of family resilience and its application in the context of family adaptation to ABI, employing a case report of a family therapy intervention to highlight key issues (Butera-Prinzi, Charles, & Story).

Two articles provide literature reviews, including a systematic scoping review examining the impact of violence-related TBIs as compared to TBIs sustained by other causes (Bates, Matthews, Simpson, & Bates) and a narrative review of the specialized literature examining the impact of TBI on a neglected yet important group, namely the siblings of people with TBI (Degeneffe). One article addresses another important aspect of community reintegration, namely the process of vocational rehabilitation and the role of informal supports in contributing to successful return to work outcomes for people with ABI (Matérne, Lundqvist, & Strandberg). The special issue is then rounded off by an important study investigating the level of workplace stress and perceived clarity of the social work role within the interdisciplinary rehabilitation team (Vungkhanching & Tonsing).

This is the largest collection of articles featuring social workers as lead authors ever produced in a single volume on the topic of TBI and ABI. The emphasis on evaluation of social work interventions is encouraging, with articles from Australia, the United States, Canada, and the United Kingdom all addressing this, given that the lack of published evaluations of practice has been identified as a significant gap in the international evidence base for the profession (Soydan, 2015). In terms of fields of practice, the articles focus largely on systemically based work with families (a key element of the social work role within the rehabilitation context; Baker, Tandy, & Dixon, 2002; Barclay, 2013; Simpson, Simons, & McFadyen, 2002), followed by approaches to different domains of community reintegration, which aim to maximize the level of participation of the person with ABI.

Brain injury rehabilitation is a specialty field for social work. Within this context, even national-based social work specialist practice groups in brain injury do not have the critical mass needed to address key challenges and exploit key opportunities for the profession within the field. Furthermore, it was critical to strengthen the presence of social workers at the highest levels within brain injury, both nationally and internationally. Social workers are good at mobilizing resources to address professional challenges, but the question arises as to how that mobilization can be achieved. Due to its specialist nature, brain injury is an issue that rarely appears on the agenda of national social work associations, nor is it a topic that has received much attention from social work academic departments around the world. However, the size and nature of the challenges are far greater than the capacity of individual practitioners, or even small groups of practitioners, to effectively address. One possible answer to this type of dilemma rests in the development of an international e-network.

The multilayered utility of e-networks has been recognized across many domains of human activity, including business, education, and social work. Dulworth (2006) highlighted that the role of "properly used networks can help improve . . . performance in a number of ways, broadening . . . exposure to new ideas and solutions and giving . . . increased access to the expertise of leaders in your field" (p. 37). With exponential growth in the access and use of communication technology, both in our personal and professional lives, online networks assist in offering opportunities to share professional knowledge and support with peers on an international scale (Macia & Garcia, 2016; Mishna, Bogo, Root, & Fantus, 2014).

INSWABI was devised to play exactly this role. INSWABI was established in 2006 at the Fifth International Conference for Social Work in Health and Mental Health in Hong Kong (Simonson & Simpson, 2010). It was the joint initiative of two special-interest practice groups, the Brain Injury Social Work Group (United Kingdom) and the Social Workers in Brain Injury Group (Australia), with both groups affiliated with their respective national social work associations. INSWABI acts as an e-network comprising approximately 130 social workers across 10 countries. The purpose of INSWABI is captured in its mission statement, which reads, "through international collaboration to enhance the social work contribution to the field for the benefit of people with acquired brain injury, their families, significant others and broader support networks" (Simonson & Simpson, 2010).

The great majority of members (approximately 90%) are practitioners, with only 5% of members holding academic or research positions. The predominant activities of INSWABI have focused on peer consultation, international exchange visits, developing resources, encouraging conference presentations, and building research capacity to expand the evidence base for social work within the field, with the last of these activities facilitated by an informal academic and practitioner mentoring approach delivered across the network, consistent with initiatives undertaking in other practice settings (e.g., Joubert & Hocking, 2015; Lunt, Ramian, Shaw, Fouché, & Mitchell, 2012). As a part of these efforts, a small number of INSWABI members have been able to continue meeting face to face at each successive triennial International Conference on Social Work in Health and Mental Health. This special issue represents another important step in developing the capacity to undertake practitioner-driven research and provide a social work voice within the field of TBI and ABI, a step that would have seemed unimaginable even 5 years ago.

Finally, in seeking to advance the contribution of social work within the field, we can continue to take inspiration from those who came before us. This is an opportunity to acknowledge the contribution of Mary Romano, a U.S. social work pioneer in the field of rehabilitation. Romano practiced in the 1970s and 1980s. She was assistant director of the Social Work Department at Columbia Presbyterian Hospital in New York, followed by the position of founding director of social work at the National Rehabilitation Hospital in Washington, DC. In addition to providing practice leadership and systems advocacy, she was active in research, sitting as a consulting editor on two journals (*Health and Social Work* and *Sexuality and Disability*), as well as publishing many articles in peer-reviewed journals about social work practice in the fields of health, rehabilitation, and disability.

One particular article authored by Romano (1974), "Family Response to Traumatic Head Injury," published in the *Scandinavian Journal of Rehabilitation Medicine*, bears special mention. As a new social worker starting in a brain injury rehabilitation unit in Sydney in the late 1980s, I [GS] found its wisdom and insights very helpful, at that stage 15 years after the article had been published. In an upcoming systematic review of all social work authored publications in the field of TBI (1970–2014), her article was the first social work authored article published in a peer-reviewed journal that we could identify. Moreover, it still remains one of the most highly cited of any articles authored by a social worker addressing the topic of TBI over the past 44 years. She died far too early, but in recognition of her contribution to the field, she was posthumously awarded the inaugural Distinguished Members Award of the American Congress of Rehabilitation Medicine in 1991. Twenty-five years later, she remains the only social work recipient of this award. Hopefully her passion, vision, and achievements can remain an inspiration to social workers in the field of rehabilitation in general, and brain injury in particular, to aspire to represent the profession at the highest levels, through the demonstration of excellence in both practice and research.

References

Access Economics. (2009). *The economic cost of spinal cord injury and traumatic brain injury in Australia*. Melbourne, Australia: Access Economics, Victorian Neurotrauma Institute.

Anderson, M. I., Simpson, G. K., & Morey, P. J. (2013). The impact of neurobehavioral impairment on family functioning and the psychological wellbeing of male versus female care-givers of relatives with severe traumatic brain injury: Multi-group analysis. *Journal of Head Trauma Rehabilitation, 28,* 453–463. doi:10.1097/htr.0b013e31825d6087

Anderson, M. I., Simpson, G. K., Morey, P. J., Mok, M. M. C., Gosling, T. J., & Gillett, L. E. (2009). Differential pathways of psychological distress in spouses versus parents of people with severe traumatic brain injury (TBI): Multi-group analysis. *Brain Injury, 23,* 931–943. doi:10.3109/02699050903302336

Anstey, K. J., Butterworth, P., Jorm, A. F., Chistensen, H., Rodgers, B., & Windsor, T. D. (2004). A population survey found an association between self-reports of traumatic brain injury and increased psychiatric symptoms. *Journal of Clinical Epidemiology, 57,* 1202–1209. doi:10.1016/j.jclinepi.2003.11.011

Australian Institute of Health and Welfare. (2007). *Disability in Australia: Acquired brain injury* (Bulletin No. 55. Cat No. AUS 96). Canberra, Australia: Author.

Baker, K. A., Tandy, C. C., & Dixon, D. R. (2002). Traumatic brain injury: A social work primer. *Journal of Social Work in Disability & Rehabilitation, 1,* 25–44. doi:10.1300/j198v01n04_03

Barclay, D. A. (2013). Family functioning, psychosocial stress, and goal attainment in brain injury rehabilitation. *Journal of Social Work in Disability & Rehabilitation, 12,* 159–175. doi:10.1080/1536710x.2013.810093

Bogner, J., & Corrigan, J. D. (2013). Interventions for substance misuse following TBI: A systematic review. *Brain Impairment, 14*(1), 77–91. doi:10.1017/brimp.2013.5

Carlton, T. O., & Stephenson, M. D. (1990). Social work and the management of severe head injury. *Social Science and Medicine, 31,* 5–11.

College of Audiologists and Speech-Language Pathologists of Ontario. (2002). *Preferred practice guideline for cognitive-communication disorders.* Toronto, ON, Canada: Author.

Dulworth, M. (2006). Enhancing personal and professional development: The role of peer networks. *Employment Relations Today, 33*(3), 37–41. doi:10.1002/ert.20116

Finkelstein, E., Corso, P. S., & Miller, T. R. (2006). *The incidence and economic burden of injuries in the United States.* New York, NY: Oxford University Press.

Frost, R. B., Farrer, T. J., Primosch, M., & Hedges, D. W. (2013). Prevalence of traumatic brain injury in the general adult population: A meta-analysis. *Neuroepidemiology, 40,* 154–159. doi:10.1159/000343275

Gould, K. R., Ponsford, J. L., Johnston, L., & Schönberger, M. (2011). Relationship between psychiatric disorders and 1-year psychosocial outcome following traumatic brain injury. *Journal of Head Trauma Rehabilitation, 26*(1), 79–89. doi:10.1097/htr.0b013e3182036799

Jennett, B., Snoek, J., Bond, M. R., & Brooks, N. (1981). Disability after severe head injury: Observations on the use of the Glasgow Outcome Scale. *Journal of Neurology, Neurosurgery & Psychiatry, 44,* 285–293. doi:10.1136/jnnp.44.4.285

Jennett, B., & Teasdale, G. (1981). *Management of head injuries.* London, UK: FA Davis.

Joubert, L., & Hocking, A. (2015). Academic practitioner partnerships: A model for collaborative practice research in social work. *Australian Social Work, 68,* 352–363. doi:10.1080/0312407x.2015.1045533

Kruetzer, J. S., Rapport, L. J., Marwitz, J. H., Harrison-Felix, C., Hart, T., Glenn, M., & Hammond, F. (2009). Caregivers' well-being after traumatic brain injury: A multicenter prospective investigation. *Archives of Physical Medicine and Rehabilitation, 90,* 939–946. doi:10.1016/j.apmr.2009.01.010

Langlois, J. A., Rutland-Brown, W., & Wald, M. W. (2006). The epidemiology and impact of traumatic brain injury: An overview. *Journal of Head Trauma Rehabilitation, 21,* 375–378. doi:10.1097/00001199-200609000-00001

Lateef, F. (2011). Bitemporal compression injury to the head. *Journal of Emergency Trauma and Shock, 4,* 411–412. doi:10.4103/0974-2700.83874

Lunt, N. T., Ramian, K., Shaw, I., Fouché, C., & Mitchell, F. (2012). Networking practitioner research: Synthesising the state of the "art". *European Journal of Social Work, 15,* 185–203. doi:10.1080/13691457.2010.513964

Macià, M., & García, I. (2016). Informal online communities and networks as a source of teacher professional development: A review. *Teaching and Teacher Education, 55,* 291–307. doi:10.1016/j.tate.2016.01.021

Menon, D. K., Schwab, K., Wright, D. W., & Maas, A. I. (2010). Demographics and clinical assessment working group of the international and interagency initiative toward common data elements for research on traumatic brain injury and psychological health: Position statement. Definition of traumatic brain injury. *Archives of Physical Medicine and Rehabilitation, 91,* 1637–1640.

Mishna, F., Bogo, M., Root, J., & Fantus, S. (2014). Here to stay: Cyber communication as a complement in social work practice. *Families in Society: The Journal of Contemporary Social Services, 95,* 179–186. doi:10.1606/1044-3894.2014.95.23

Oddy, M., Moir, J. F., Fortescue, D., & Chadwick, S. (2012). The prevalence of traumatic brain injury in the homeless community in a UK city. *Brain Injury, 26,* 1058–1064. doi:10.3109/02699052.2012.667595

Peeters, W., van den Brande, R., Polinder, S., Brazinova, A., Steyerberg, E. W., Lingsma, H. F., & Maas, A. I. (2015). Epidemiology of traumatic brain injury in Europe. *Acta Neurochirurgica, 157*, 1683–1696. doi:10.1007/s00701–015–2512–7

Perlesz, A., Kinsella, G., & Crowe, S. (1999). Impact of traumatic brain injury on the family: A critical review. *Rehabilitation Psychology, 44*(1), 6–35. doi:10.1037/0090–5550.44.1.6

Ponsford, J. L., Downing, M. G., Olver, J., Ponsford, M., Acher, R., Carty, M., & Spitz, G. (2014). Longitudinal follow-up of patients with traumatic brain injury: Outcome at two, five, and ten years post-injury. *Journal of Neurotrauma, 31*(1), 64–77. doi:10.1089/neu.2013.2997

Ponsford, J. L., Janzen, S., McIntyre, A., Bayley, M., Velikonja, D., & Tate, R. (2014). INCOG recommendations for management of cognition following traumatic brain injury: Part I. Posttraumatic amnesia/delirium. *Journal of Head Trauma Rehabilitation, 29,* 307–320. doi:10.1097/htr.0000000000000074

Ponsford, J. L., Sloan, S., & Snow, P. (2013). *Traumatic brain injury: Rehabilitation for everyday adaptive living* (2nd ed.). Hove, UK: Psychology Press.

Romano, M. D. (1974). Family response to traumatic head injury. *Scandinavian Journal of Rehabilitation Medicine, 6*(1), 1–4.

Rona, R. J., Jones, M., Fear, N. T., Hull, L., Murphy, D., Machell, L., . . . Greenberg, N. (2012). Mild traumatic brain injury in UK military personnel returning from Afghanistan and Iraq: Cohort and cross-sectional analyses. *The Journal of Head Trauma Rehabilitation, 27,* 33–44. doi:10.1097/htr.0b013e318212f814

Rowlands, A. (2000). Understanding social support and friendship: Implications for intervention after acquired brain injury. *Brain Impairment, 1,* 151–164. doi:10.1375/brim.1.2.151

Russell, W. R., & Smith, A. (1961). Post-traumatic amnesia in closed head injury. *Archives of Neurology, 5,* 4–17. doi:10.1001/archneur.1961.00450130006002

Sabaz, M., Simpson, G. K., Walker, A. J., Rogers, J. M., Gillis, I., & Strettles, B. (2014). Prevalence, co-morbidities and predictors of challenging behavior among a cohort of community-dwelling adults with severe traumatic brain injury: A multi-center study. *Journal of Head Trauma Rehabilitation, 29,* E19–E30. doi:10.1097/htr.0b013e31828dc590

Sander, A. M., Sherer, M., Malec, J. F., High, W. M., Jr., Thompson, R. N., Moessner, A. M., & Josey, J. (2003). Preinjury emotional and family functioning in caregivers of persons with traumatic brain injury. *Archives of Physical Medicine and Rehabilitation, 84,* 197–203. doi:10.1053/apmr.2003.50105

Simonson, P., & Simpson, K. (2010, June–July). *Building international networks to promote social work practice in specialty fields: The experience of the international network for social workers in acquired brain injury.* Presentation at Changing Health: 6th International Conference on Social Work in Health and Mental Health, University College Dublin, Dublin, Ireland.

Simpson, G., & Jones, K. (2013). How important is resilience among family members supporting relatives with traumatic brain injury or spinal cord injury? *Clinical Rehabilitation, 27,* 367–377. doi:10.1177/0269215512457961

Simpson, G., Simons, M., & McFadyen, M. (2002). The challenges of a hidden disability: Social work practice in the field of traumatic brain injury. *Australian Social Work, 55,* 24–37. doi:10.1080/03124070208411669

Simpson, G., & Tate, R. (2007). Suicidality in people surviving a traumatic brain injury: Prevalence, risk factors and implications for clinical management. *Brain Injury, 21,* 1335–1351. doi:10.1080/02699050701785542

Soydan, H. (2015). Intervention research in social work. *Australian Social Work, 68,* 324–337. doi:10.1080/0312407x.2014.993670

Tate, R. L., McDonald, S., & Lulham, J. M. (1998). Incidence of hospital treated traumatic brain injury in an Australian community. *Australian and New Zealand Journal of Public Health, 22,* 419–423. doi:10.1111/j.1467–842x.1998.tb01406.x

Tate, R. L., Simpson, G. K., & McRae, P. (2015). Traumatic brain injury. In R. Escorpizo, S. Brage, D. Homa, & G. Stucki (Eds.), *Handbook of vocational rehabilitation and disability evaluation: Application and implementation of the ICF* (pp. 263–294). New York, NY: Springer.

Teasdale, G. M. (1995). Head injury. *Journal of Neurology, Neurosurgery, and Psychiatry, 58,* 526–539.

Teasdale, G. M., & Jennett, B. (1974). Assessment of coma and impaired consciousness: A practical scale. *Lancet, 13*(2), 81–84.

Tsaousides, T., Ashman, T. A., & Gordon, W. A. (2013). Diagnosis and treatment of depression following traumatic brain injury. *Brain Impairment, 14,* 63–76. doi:10.1017/brimp.2013.8

Tyerman, A. (2012). Vocational rehabilitation after traumatic brain injury: Models and services. *NeuroRehabilitation, 31,* 51–62. doi:10.3233/NRE–2012–0774

Williams, W. H., Mewse, A. J., Tonks, J., Mills, S., Burgess, C. N. W., & Cordan, G. (2010). Traumatic brain injury in a prison population: Prevalence and risk for re-offending. *Brain Injury, 24,* 1184–1188. doi:10.3109/02699052.2010.495697

Wood, R. L., & Yurdakul, L. K. (1997). Change in relationship status following traumatic brain injury. *Brain Injury, 11,* 491–501. doi:10.1080/bij.11.7.491.501

Family Forward: Promoting Family Adaptation Following Pediatric Acquired Brain Injury

Lyndal Hickey, Vicki Anderson, and Brigid Jordan

ABSTRACT
This article describes a new and innovative social work intervention, Family Forward, designed to promote early adaptation of the family system after the onset of a child's acquired brain injury. Family Forward is integrated into inpatient rehabilitation services provided to the injured child and recognizes the important role of family in child rehabilitation outcomes and the parallel process of recovery for the child and family following an injury. Family Forward is informed by clinical practice, existing research in family adaptation after pediatric acquired brain injury, the resiliency model of family adjustment and adaptation, and family therapy theories and approaches.

Acquired brain injury (ABI) can result from a number of causes after birth, including trauma, hypoxia stroke, infections, neurological disorders, and tumors. An ABI can cause physical, cognitive, psychosocial, and sensory impairments, which could lead to restrictions in various areas of life (Australian Institute of Health & Welfare, 2007). Pediatric ABI is often sudden and unexpected; families are unprepared to deal with issues surrounding the injury, subsequent hospitalization, and reintegration into the home. A child's injury can be experienced as a psychological trauma to the whole family system. It is a period of crisis and disruption for families as they support the child throughout the acute and rehabilitation phases of care while striving to meet the needs of all family members.

Rehabilitation outcomes for children with ABI are closely associated with family functioning and capacity to meet the changing needs of the injured child over time (Lax Pericall & Taylor, 2014; Ryan et al., 2015; Schmidt, Orsten, Hanten, Li, & Levin, 2010; Taylor et al., 1995; Yeates, Taylor, Walz, Stancin, & Wade, 2010; Ylvisaker et al., 2005). Families experience substantial stress and burden, depression, psychological distress, and economic disadvantage in the first 12 months following a child's injury (Conoley & Sheridan, 1996; Gan, Campbell, Gemeinhardt, & McFadden, 2006; Stancin, Wade, Walz, Yeates, & Taylor, 2008; Wade, Michaud, & Brown, 2006; Wade, Taylor, et al.,

2006; Wade et al., 2001). It is therefore vital for rehabilitation services to develop effective ways of working with families during the early stages postinjury to maximize outcomes for the child.

The social work scope of practice within pediatric rehabilitation services is to provide psychosocial interventions to assist families during the child's inpatient and ambulatory rehabilitation. Despite the recognition in the literature of the importance of families in child rehabilitation outcomes, there is limited research about effective psychosocial interventions to promote family adaptation following the early stages postinjury (Conoley & Sheridan, 1996; Gan et al., 2006; Wade et al., 1996). Currently, there is no evidence base for effective social work interventions with families during a child's inpatient rehabilitation phase of care.

Family Forward is currently under trial in a pediatric inpatient service at the Royal Children's Hospital in Melbourne, Australia. It is a response to the clinical and research gap about how social workers best meet the psychosocial needs of families during a child's inpatient phase of care and transition to home. The evaluation of this intervention will contribute to ABI research and inform future social work rehabilitation practices with families as they embark on a process of adaptation parallel to their child's recovery from injury.

This article outlines important contributions to the development of Family Forward, including research knowledge on family adaptation for pediatric ABI, a definition of family adaptation that reflects the family experience after ABI, and family therapy as a conceptual framework and practice approach. Family Forward is described using themes derived from the family adaptation definition of the resiliency model of family adjustment and adaptation (H. I. McCubbin, Thompson, & McCubbin, 1996; M. A. McCubbin, McCubbin, Danielson, Hamel-Bissell, & Winstead-Fry, 1993).

Family adaptation

The Family Forward design has been informed by research in the area of family adaptation following pediatric ABI. The research to date has defined the adaptation process using one or two constructs such as family functioning, family burden and distress, parent coping, and predictors of family outcomes (Stancin et al., 2008; Wade, Taylor, et al., 2006; Wade et al., 1996). Quantitative studies have focused on child and family outcomes, whereas qualitative studies have explored the impact on family relationships. All relevant studies that have informed Family Forward are summarized in Table 1.

Family functioning has a significant influence on child and family outcomes. Aspects of family functioning that might alter as a result of the child's ABI are division of day-to-day tasks, communication patterns, the amount and quality of time spent with various family members, and limit setting with

Table 1. Family adaptation.

Study	Participants	Family outcome measures	Main findings related to family adaptation
Ryan et al. (2015)	N = 118 (TBI n = 78, control n = 40)	Family Burden of Injury Interview (FBII), Family Assessment Device (FAD)	1. Poor long-term social outcomes were associated with poor family functioning and poorer caregiver mental health. 2. Clinician-delivered, family-centered interventions might assist caregivers to mobilize more adaptive coping.
Sambuco et al. (2012)	N = 39 Siblings closest in age to a child with moderate or severe TBI	Social Support Scale for Children The Family Adaptability and Cohesion Evaluation Scales II	1. Reduced self-esteem in siblings. 2. No behavioral difficulties in siblings. 3. Sibling knowledge of TBI and social support associated with behavioral outcomes.
Wade et al. (2010)	N = 48 TBI (severe TBI n = 11, moderate TBI n = 37) N = 89 orthopedic injury Families of children age 3–6 years	FBII Brief Symptom Inventory (BSI) COPE	1. Mothers were more likely than fathers to cope regardless of the nature or severity of injury. 2. Fathers more likely to use denial to cope following TBI. 3. Mothers of children with TBI experienced elevated levels of burden and distress compared with mothers in orthopedic injury group. 4. Fathers reported greater injury-related stress and distress than mothers over time.
Stancin et al. (2008)	N = 89 TBI (severe TBI n = 21, moderate TBI n = 22, complicated mild TBI n = 46) N = 117 orthopedic injury Families of children age 3–6 years	Family Assessment Device (FAD–GF) Life Stressors and Social Resources Inventory (LISRES-A) FBII BSI	1. Families generally adapted well. 2. TBI groups marginally more adversely affected than orthopedic injury group. 3. Severe and complicated mild TBI groups had greater overall injury-related stress, psychological distress, and depressive symptoms. 4. Chronic life stressors and interpersonal resources are determinants of injury and distress. 5. Use of denial and avoidant coping strategies associated with elevated burden and distress. 6. Burden and distress moderated by child's age at injury. Severe TBI in older children associated with greater injury-related burden.
Clark et al. (2008)	N = 10 Mothers of children (0–16 years) with ABI (2–10 years) postinjury.	Interview	1. Relationship changes associated with child's change in personality and temperament. 2. Mother: posttrauma symptoms present; difficulties in processing emotional response; permanency of injury; change in role definition. 3. Family changes: Short-term increase in protectiveness, closeness; and isolated. Long-term negotiating greater independence between family members. 4. Parents described minimal ABI information, difficulties in absorbing information at the time of child's injury.

(Continued)

Table 1. Continued.

Study	Participants	Family outcome measures	Main findings related to family adaptation
Catroppa, Anderson, Morse, Haritou, and Rosenfeld (2008)	N = 65 (severe TBI n = 15, moderate TBI n = 22, mild TBI n = 11) Control (healthy) n = 17	Family Functioning Scale (FFQ) FBII and socioeconomic status (SES)	1. Moderate TBI group largest discrepancy from preinjury to 5 years postinjury, with a suggestion of poorer family functioning at 5 years postinjury.
Wade, Taylor, et al. (2006)	N = 168 (severe TBI n = 46 moderate TBI n = 54 and orthopedic injury n = 68) Families of children with TBI and orthopedic injury	SCI LISRES-A FBII BSI FAD–GF	1. Decline in carer burden across follow-up intervals of all groups moderated by resources. 2. Severe TBI group had higher injury-related burden than the other two groups. 3. Higher burden and distress in moderate TBI to orthopedic injury group. Burden and distress declined over time. 4. Severe TBI associated with some long-term burden but adequate interpersonal resources reduce risk.
Robson et al. (2005)	N = 6 Parents of children (2–15 years) with TBI 6 months postdischarge	Semistructured interviews	1. Emotional response to transitioning home with injured child more challenging than physical care. 2. Different family member responses to transitioning home resulted in increased stress; disproportionate burden placed on mothers. 3. Support from close relationships and coping strategies promotes adjustment of family members after injury.
Benn and McColl (2004)	N = 30 Parents of children child with ABI (up to 2 years) postinjury	Ways of Coping Questionnaire (face-to-face I/V) Interpersonal Support Evaluation List Family Environment Scale (FES)	1. Most common parent coping strategies were perception-focused coping. 2. Mothers had larger coping repertoire than fathers using more strategies more often. 3. Maternal and paternal coping were complementary in nature. 4. Relationship between instrumental (practical) support and emotion-focused coping. 5. Relationship between family cohesion and perception-focused coping.
Wade et al. (2003)	N = 82 (severe TBI n = 25, moderate TBI, n = 22, and orthopedic injury n = 35) Parents and adolescents with TBI and orthopedic injury	Observer parent–child interactions Conflict Behaviour Questionnaire, FBII, BSI, and FAD	1. No group differences on ratings of parent–adolescent interaction. 2. Severe TBI group observed criticism and coldness and self-rated conflict had stronger associations with injury-related stress, caregiver distress, and family functioning.
Wade et al. (2002)	N = 189 (severe TBI n = 53, moderate TBI n = 56, and orthopedic injury n = 80) Parents of children with TBI and orthopedic injury	SCI LISRES-A FBII BSI FAD–GF	1. TBI groups did not report higher levels of caregiver psychological distress or family dysfunction than orthopedic injury group. 2. Severe TBI group had greater injury-related stress and burden, deterioration in preinjury levels of family function 6 months after injury, and a subsequent improvement in family functioning from 6 to 12 months relative to the other two groups. 3. Decrease in injury-related stress and burden. 4. Favorable adaptation for most families.

Study	Sample	Measures	Findings
Anderson et al. (2001)	N = 112 (severe n = 29, moderate n = 52, mild n = 31) Parents of children age 2–12 years with TBI	SES FFQ FBII	1. Family functioning stable preinjury to 6 months postinjury. 2. Although no change in family functioning, severe TBI group had higher levels of burden and stress. 3. No clear relationship between levels of family functioning, injury severity, age at injury, and physical or cognitive disability.
Wade et al. (2001)	N = 174 (TBI n = 103 and orthopedic injury n = 71) Families of children TBI and orthopedic injury	SCI LISRES-A COPE FBII BSI FAD–GF	1. Partial support emotion-focused coping strategies associated with more favorable caregiver and family outcomes. 2. Denial and disengagement associated with more adverse outcomes such as carer psychological distress. 3. Injury acceptance associated with lower burden and denial in both TBI and orthopedic injury groups.
Max et al. (1998)	N = 50 Children with TBI (6–14 years)	McMaster Structured Interview of Family Functioning, FAD Interview: preinjury family functioning, Family Life Events (FILE)	1. Lack of significance of "novel" or "never before present" psychiatric disorder on family function at 3 months. 2. Psychopathology in children after TBI relates to postinjury family functioning, taking into account preinjury family functioning. 3. Unclear whether new psychopathology induces deterioration in family functioning or vice versa.
Wade et al. (1998)	N = 189 (severe TBI n = 53, moderate TBI n = 56, orthopedic injury n = 80)	SCI LISRES-A FBII BSI and FAD–GF	1. Severe TBI group had persistent carer stress associated with child's injury; relative risk of clinically significant psychological symptoms (nearly twice that of orthopedic injury group).
Rivara et al. (1996)	N = 81 families of children (6–15 years) with ABI and loss of consciousness	FES, FAD, FILE, Health Insurance Survey – general well being Family Global Assessment Scale Family Interview Rating Scale	1. Preinjury functioning was best predictor of outcomes. 2. Fewer changes in family functioning reported over 3 years in mild and moderate groups. 3. 33% to 50% of parents in moderate or severe groups reported medium to high strain. 4. Severe TBI had positive change associated with better preinjury levels of communication, expressiveness, problem solving, use of resources, role flexibility, greater activity orientation, and less conflict, control, and stress.

Note: TBI = traumatic brain injury; ABI = acquired brain injury.

the injured child (Wade, Drotar, Taylor, & Stancin, 1995). Longitudinal studies up to 6 years postinjury have found most families make the necessary adaptations to care for the injured child and restore family functioning with some variability related to injury severity (Anderson et al., 2001; Catroppa, Anderson, Morse, Haritou, & Rosenfeld, 2008; Ryan et al., 2015; Wade, Taylor, et al., 2006). Nevertheless some families have reported some deterioration in family functioning in the first 12 months postinjury, particularly evident in families caring for a child with a severe injury (Robson, Ziviani, & Spina, 2005; Wade et al., 2003). The majority of children with severe ABI are admitted to inpatient rehabilitation services during this period and tailoring interventions to alleviate challenges for this group was a key consideration for the design of the intervention described in this article. Similarly, the intervention needed to take into account key findings from the qualitative literature to assist families' transition to home and to promote positive patterns of family interaction and relationships.

Family functioning is also associated with the development of psychopathology in the injured child in the first 24 months postinjury (Max et al., 1998). In a qualitative study conducted with families transitioning their child from hospital to home, changes to the spousal relationship and parent–child dyad with noninjured siblings were also noted. Families attributed these changes to the stresses associated with the child's injury and prolonged periods of separation. The relationship between the parent and injured child was also affected, with parents experiencing an increased level of protection toward the child and reluctance to separate (Robson et al., 2005). Mothers interviewed several years after their child's injury report changes in family functioning as a response to the behavioral problems of the injured child (Clark, Stedmon, & Margison, 2008).

The identification of predictors of child and family outcomes also provide important insights for how Family Forward tailors interventions and targets resources for families during the rehabilitation phase of care. Pre and post family functioning, which includes family cohesion, good communication, and better coping resources, have been found to be reliable predictors for positive child and family outcomes postinjury (Anderson et al., 2001; Max et al., 1998; Rivara et al., 1996; Stancin et al., 2008; Wade, Michaud, et al., 2006). Predictors of negative family outcomes are associated with family members' premorbid psychiatric health and general health, families with poorly functioning households, fewer coping skills, anxiety and depression, and higher levels of stress (Max et al., 1998; Rivara et al., 1996). Chronic life stressors and interpersonal resources are also predictors of families experiencing injury burden and distress (Stancin et al., 2008; Wade, Michaud, et al., 2006), and there is a relationship between the predictors of psychosocial outcomes such as the injured child's behavior, family functioning, and family burden. The injured child's problematic postinjury behavior is associated with his or her preinjury behavior, increased care related to physical impairment, and family difficulties postinjury (Anderson et al., 2001).

Studies focusing on family burden, stress, and psychological distress report that families with children with ABI are more adversely affected compared with families of children with orthopedic injuries, although the differences are small (Stancin et al., 2008; Wade, Michaud, et al., 2006; Wade, Taylor, Drotar, Stancin, & Yeates, 1998, 2002). Severity of injury is also a factor in the level of stress and burden experienced by families. Families of children with severe or complicated mild injuries report greater overall stress compared with the moderate TBI and orthopedic cohorts (Anderson et al., 2001; Stancin et al., 2008).

The time lapsed since injury is also a consideration. Wade and colleagues have reported that families of children with severe TBI experience far greater stress and burden at 12 months, with a deterioration in preinjury levels of family function at 6 months and a subsequent improvement from 6 to 12 months relative to other groups (Wade et al., 2002). Several years on, families reported a decline in carer burden and stress moderated by interpersonal resources (Stancin et al., 2008; Wade et al., 1998; Wade, Taylor, et al., 2006). The findings of elevated burden and stress are important considerations for Family Forward as similar to the family functioning research; families identified at risk of increased burden and stress in the first 12 months are those with children with severe TBI, and this cohort is typically admitted for inpatient rehabilitation services.

Coping is another construct employed in research to understand the family adaptation process. Studies have defined the positive and negative impacts of coping on adaptation in relation to family cohesion, optimism, participation in recreational activities, and the subjective meaning parents give to the experience (Benn & McColl, 2004; Martin, 1988; Wade et al., 2001; Wade et al., 2010). Parents reporting positive coping tended to use strategies that altered their perception of the child's injury; experienced differences in maternal and paternal coping as complementary; and employed emotion-oriented strategies to deal with their changed circumstance (Benn & McColl, 2004; Wade et al., 2001). Differences in coping within families can prove problematic for family adaptation, particularly in the initial period postinjury. Coping challenges have also been reported in the areas of learning about the child's ABI, the increased amount of care for the injured child, the emotional impact, and accessing appropriate resources (Gan, Gargaro, Brandys, Gerber, & Boschen, 2010).

Family Forward has sought to understand ways in which parental coping can be optimized to integrate the key findings of this research into the intervention. Tensions arising in the spousal relationship can often be resolved quickly when mediated by an external family member or health professional, with the resolution located in the recognition and acceptance of different coping styles of each parent by the other (Robson et al., 2005). Professional counseling to assist parents to recognize positive coping strategies can result in a reduction of family stress and dysfunction over time (Benn & McColl, 2004; Wade et al., 2001). Conversely, families who employ negative coping strategies such as denial or other avoidant ways of coping in the early stages postinjury have reported long-term tensions in the spousal relationship (Clark et al., 2008; Stancin et al., 2008). Parental denial and disengagement following a child's injury can often indicate the emergence of acute stress disorder or is indicative of a personality style lacking in adequate coping skills (Stancin et al., 2008). In a qualitative study by Clark et al. (2008), several mothers attributed their posttrauma responses several years after their child's injury to a lack of processing of the emotional experiences surrounding the injury shortly after the event.

There are numerous methodological limitations in current research, such as different constructs defined and measured as family adaptation and lack of clarity in the psychosocial interventions delivered to families involved in the studies. The studies also have small sample sizes and heterogeneity in child and family demographics. In spite of these limitations, the research provides important insights for Family Forward into the impact of pediatric ABI on family functioning, factors that influence child and family outcomes, and key aspects of family adaptation.

Family therapy

Family Forward has conceptualized the family experience following pediatric ABI using family therapy theory and approaches. Family therapy is a broad term that describes a range of theories and approaches for working with families experiencing problems or challenges. Family therapy theories of most relevance to this article view the family as a system that functions and maintains a homeostasis or balance using established rules, family roles, and communication styles; recurring patterns of interaction; and negotiating differences between members for the development and well-being of its members (Carr, 2012). Families that function well are successful at balancing the needs of individual members and the family system as a whole. The meanings, understandings, and assumptions a family makes about the world reflect the narratives and stories it has created about itself (Cavallo & Kay, 2005; Goldenberg & Goldenberg, 2013; Maitz & Sachs, 1995).

Family therapy has developed different concepts for understanding and promoting change in the family system. Key concepts applicable to families of children with ABI during the early stages of recovery include the following:
- Focusing on the present and appraising how immediate, ongoing interactions and sequences between family members affect the family system's ability to adapt.

- Gathering and interpreting information about the family system located within the different meanings each person within the family gives to the event or situation.
- Reducing symptomatic issues that are problematic.
- Increasing family members' level of differentiation to improve the ability of the system to adapt.
- Providing education so the family can develop skills and coping to meet the changed needs of its members.
- Supporting family members as they manage the consequences associated with adaptive changes within the system.

Family therapy conceptualizes a child's ABI as a disruption to the homeostasis and functioning of the family system. Family adaptation requires the family system to reestablish a new homeostasis postinjury to meet the changing needs of its members. An injury to the child is an injury to the family system and therefore the recovery process for the child and family need to run parallel for optimal adaptation to occur (Cavallo & Kay, 2005). The family adaptation process has also been described as families needing to undertake four tasks: the task of grieving, the task of restructuring, the task of developing a new identity, and the task of growing through adversity (Perlesz, Furlong, & McLachlan, 1992). Other conceptual frameworks include the family system recovery process moving through six stages: optimism during the hospitalization; bewilderment and anxiety when the family returns home with the injured member; feelings of guilt; depression, despair, and mourning; reorganization; and emotional disengagement (Lezak, 1986).

Family therapists have argued that family therapy is unlikely to be effective in the early stages following an ABI (Aitken et al., 2004; Laroi, 2003; Perlesz et al., 1992). However, family therapy concepts can be woven through Family Forward and guide the social worker's practice and assist families in understanding the system changes that are occurring in their family. The social work profession also derives many aspects of practice from family systems theory and is able to incorporate family therapy approaches and skills with families. Social work within pediatric rehabilitation services is well placed to provide interventions that integrate social work and family therapy into a rehabilitation response to the child's injury.

Resiliency model of family adjustment and adaptation

Family Forward uses the resiliency model of family stress, adjustment and adaptation (H. I. McCubbin et al., 1996; M. A. McCubbin et al., 1993) to define the process of family adjustment adaptation (see Figure 1). According to the resiliency model, families negotiate change brought about by stressful events and situations with an innate ability to maintain stability and

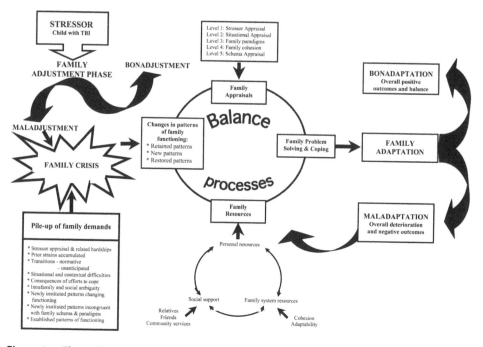

Figure 1. The resiliency model family stress, adjustment, and adaptation phase for families of children with a traumatic brain injury. Adapted from McCubbin, Thompson, and McCubbin (1996). Reproduced with permission from Cambridge University Press: Spina et al. (2005).

established patterns of behavior. Family adjustment is characterized by relatively minor changes in the family system in response to a stressor. Family adaptation occurs when many stressors culminate into a crisis, requiring families to make more substantial changes to existing patterns of functioning to reorganize and achieve a new balance over time.

The resiliency model provides a broader definition than those used in previous studies for understanding the family adaptation process following pediatric brain injury and the subsequent transitions experienced by families over time (Carnes & Quinn, 2005; Kosciulek, McCubbin, & McCubbin, 1993; Rivara et al., 1992; Rivara et al., 1996; Spina, Ziviani, & Nixon, 2005).

Family Forward has integrated this definition into themes explored with families to understand their experience and promote early adaptation. During the early stages of recovery and the rehabilitation phase of care, common family stressors relate to dealing with uncertainty of the child's prognosis, changes in the roles of family members, prolonged periods of separation, financial strain through loss of income, and any additional costs associated with hospitalization. Families respond to the stressor in the initial stages of a child's hospitalization by making changes, such as alternate child care for siblings or reduction or cessation of work commitments. Once the child's survival is assured and the recovery process begins, the magnitude of the stressor is likely to evoke a crisis for the family system, resulting in a move to the adaptation phase of the resiliency model. This adaptation phase enables the family to make more significant changes to adequately respond to the cumulative and chronic stressors associated with the child's injury recovery.

In addition to a range of preexisting stressors that a family might bring to the situation, there can also be stressors relating to the child's lengthy rehabilitation, the uncertainty of recovery, the trauma surrounding the event that led to the child's injury, guilt associated with the acquired nature of the injury, and grief for their previously healthy child. According to the resiliency model, the degree to which the family adapts will depend on a range of resiliency factors including family resources, the meaning they attribute to the situation, family coping processes, and problem-solving abilities (H. I. McCubbin et al., 1996; M. A. McCubbin et al., 1993). These factors are the foundation for Family Forward.

Family forward

Social work services in Australian pediatric rehabilitation services focus on psychosocial interventions with children and their families within a multidisciplinary or interdisciplinary team approach. Current social work practice conceptualizes the child's rehabilitation using a biopsychosocial framework, responding to presenting issues that are identified by the family or rehabilitation team using a referral process (Zittel, Lawrence, & Wodarski, 2002). Rehabilitation goals are developed with the child and family and reviewed on a regular basis. These goals are often focused on the recovery of the child as an individual and his or her participation at home, at school, and in the community.

Family Forward locates the child's recovery within family recovery and promotes "holistic" family adaptation. The intervention commences when the child is admitted to inpatient rehabilitation and the goals are integrated into the child's overall rehabilitation plan. A trial is currently underway of Family Forward. An evaluation of the intervention will contribute toward clinical and research knowledge in social work and rehabilitation practices in this area.

Family Forward is proactive and seeks to normalize the family experience of crisis postinjury and encourage the family system to move toward adaptation. Family Forward is designed for delivery by social workers within a pediatric rehabilitation service. The social worker works systemically with the family and rehabilitation team to ensure both systems are working in concert to maximize child rehabilitation outcomes. This systemic practice extends beyond the rehabilitation service to external systems and services in the community.

Long periods of separation are common for families when a child with ABI is hospitalized. Although it is often not possible to have all family members present for the intervention sessions throughout the child's inpatient rehabilitation stay, the family system is kept in mind. This is achieved by bringing the perspective of absent family members into the discussion being addressed in the session. Sessions with the injured child's siblings are offered to the family to ensure that their needs are being met during the inpatient rehabilitation stay and to prepare them for the return of the injured child to the family home.

The structure of Family Forward includes counseling and multifamily groups.

Counseling

The social worker delivers two family counseling sessions per week throughout the child's inpatient rehabilitation admission. Sessions are introduced to families as an integral part of the child's rehabilitation process with knowledge that some of the issues discussed in the sessions will be shared with the rehabilitation team if relevant to the child's rehabilitation plan. The sessions cover a range of themes identified in the literature as optimizing family adaptation and are underpinned by relevant family therapy concepts. The counseling sessions are made available to all family members affected by the child's injury. Wherever possible, siblings are included in these sessions.

Multifamily groups

Multifamily groups are offered once a week for families who have a child as an inpatient or up to the first 6 weeks postdischarge. The sessions have a psychoeducational focus and explore the following topics: injury to the child is an injury to the family, siblings, trauma and grief responses, injury recovery and rehabilitation, managing stress and coping, resources to help your family, carer self-care, and going home. The group sessions are designed as stand-alone topics as group membership is open. The total number of sessions that families attend might differ depending on the length of the child's inpatient stay and his or her ability to return as an outpatient.

Family forward adaptation themes

The family adaptation themes are integrated into the family and multifamily group sessions delivered by the social worker. The themes provide a broader definition of family adaptation outlined in the resiliency model (H. I. McCubbin et al., 1996; M. A. McCubbin et al., 1993) and provide a framework for conceptualizing and informing the intervention. The themes provide a conceptual framework for the Family Forward assessment and intervention and can be tailored to meet the unique needs of each family. Theses themes are summarized in Table 2.

Table 2. Summary of family forward assessment and interventions.

Resiliency model	Family forward assessment and interventions	Family forward mode of service delivery
Crisis	Commencement of psychosocial assessment. Assess family response to initial crisis. Handover from acute social worker. Define family description of ABI event and experience of child's acute phase of care. Appraise family system changes and adjustments during acute phase of care. Review and plan further family system changes and adjustments in preparation of rehabilitation phase of care.	Handover from acute social worker Inpatient rehabilitation services Family counseling Liaise with internal and external service providers Integration into child's rehabilitation plan
Pile-up of demands	Identify family predictive factors and possible impact on family adaptation outcomes. Identify preexisting family stressors and family system coping strategies. Assess general health and well-being of all family members. Develop self-care plan for family members to promote health and well-being.	Family counseling Referral to external service providers
Changes in family patterns	Identify preinjury family functioning, roles, tasks, and routines. Reestablish and redefine family roles, tasks, and routines. Focus on sibling(s) inclusion and engagement in process of family system change. Prepare postinjury family functioning.	Family counseling Multifamily group work
Family appraisal	Appraise experience of ABI event in relation to grief response, trauma, and perceptions of injury. Provide trauma and grief psychoeducation and information.	Family counseling Multifamily group work Liaise with internal and external service providers
Family problem solving and coping	Problem solve and negotiate care responsibilities. Acknowledge positive coping strategies and modify negative coping strategies. Identify individual and family system needs. Appraise current met and unmet needs and anticipate future needs. Develop a plan to meet current and future needs. Monitor psychological distress and refer to specialist services as clinically indicated.	Family counseling Multifamily group work Liaise with internal and external service providers
Family resources	Identify resources needed for family system to care for child in the community.	Multifamily group work Liaise with internal and external service providers

(Continued)

Table 2. Continued.

Resiliency model	Family forward assessment and interventions	Family forward mode of service delivery
	Appraise current informal family supports and changed care needs of the injured child.	
	Identify formal supports and collaboration on the completion of referrals.	
	Provide ABI psychoeducation and information.	
Family adaptation	Review of psychosocial assessment.	Ambulatory rehabilitation services
	Define family description of child's community reintegration and experience of child's care at home.	Integration into child's rehabilitation plan
		Family counseling
	Appraise family system changes and early adaptation during child's community reintegration.	Multifamily group work
		Liaise with internal and external service providers
	Review and plan further family system changes and adaptations.	Handover to community-based rehabilitation services
	Monitor engagement with informal and formal supports and referrals.	
	Discharge to community-based rehabilitation services.	

Note: ABI = acquired brain injury.

Family crisis and pile-up of demands

The crisis associated with the child's injury and subsequent hospitalization marks the beginning of the adaptation process for the family. The family enters the rehabilitation service with their child and Family Forward commences. Family Forward seeks to understand the family's experience and perceptions of events that led to the child's ABI and subsequent acute hospitalization. This process enables the social worker to assess how the family system has responded to the crisis and the changes that have already occurred to family functioning, providing important insights into how the family system has adjusted to date. The child's transition to inpatient rehabilitation is an opportune time for the social worker and family to review whether the changes that have been made to the family system are assisting them to adjust or if further modifications are required to optimize family functioning for the duration of the rehabilitation admission.

Preexisting stressors experienced by families are also explored by the social worker as part of the initial assessment of the predictive factors that might affect adaptation and recovery outcomes for the child and family. This information will assist the social worker and family to identify appropriate formal and informal interventions and resources required to alleviate the negative impact of these stressors. Family Forward acknowledges the magnitude of the crisis associated with the child's injury and the family's strengths and abilities in making necessary adjustments to manage the child's admission in the short term. The social worker also prepares the family for more substantial change that will be sustained over time by defining the process of family adaptation as family recovery.

Changes in family patterns

Family Forward incorporates an understanding of preinjury family functioning and preparing the family system for postinjury family functioning. Preinjury family functioning assists with the identification of predictors that will affect the family system's ability to adapt to the child's changed needs. The exploration of the preinjury family functioning is intended to highlight and optimize positive adaptive skills and abilities, address symptomatic issues that might be problematic, and target appropriate resources accordingly.

The division of tasks is typically assigned to roles within the family system. Family Forward assists the family to identify preinjury roles and subsequent changes to these roles in response to the child's injury. Families identify existing roles and tasks that can be maintained, make decisions about how new roles will be assigned, and review the division of tasks for the family to adapt to its changed circumstances and reestablish a new homeostasis. The spousal system in particular is examined to ensure that roles are assigned so that one parent is not overburdened.

The sibling relationship is included in the conceptualization of the family system recovery. Sibling relationships are a significant familial relationship over a person's lifetime. Siblings have significant developmental importance to one another. The resources of the family system are often relocated to focus on the injured child's hospital stay and rehabilitation, with long periods of separation of family members. As a result, siblings might be faced with changes to family routines, changes in family structure and roles, decreased emotional and physical availability of parents, and increased stress related to caregiving responsibilities. Family Forward encourages families to explore the impact on siblings and engage them in the family recovery process to optimize sibling behavioral outcomes (Sambuco, Brookes, Catroppa, & Lah, 2012).

Parents often find it challenging to leave the child's bedside in the early stages of rehabilitation, making it difficult for them to reconnect with their spouse the and noninjured siblings. Family Forward explores strategies to assist parents in meeting the needs of their injured child, while tolerating time away to reconnect with other family members and reorient themselves to life at home. This is an important preparative step for families as they ready themselves to care for their child at home. Developing short-term routines that promote engagement with family members can also return parents to their executive role of organizing and providing some predictability and assurance for noninjured siblings. Family Forward encourages families to consider ways of configuring their roles and responsibilities in the family that restore and maintain key aspects of family member routines wherever possible during the rehabilitation phase of care.

Family Forward also addresses communication patterns of the family. Family members increase awareness of their communication patterns within the family system but also with the interface of other systems, such as the rehabilitation team. The aim of this intervention is to identify communication patterns that support family members to foster positive interactions and address problematic issues as they arise. Family Forward also builds family capacity to develop their communication approach with the service system, resolve problems with service providers, and navigate their way through the service system.

Family appraisal

Family Forward supports families to appraise and attribute meaning to the events surrounding their child's injury. The appraisal focuses on three aspects of the family experience: grief response, trauma, and perceptions of the child's injury. It seeks to assist family members to understand their individual experiences and the impact of the child's injury on the family as a whole.

The grief associated with the child's ABI is acknowledged with the family in Family Forward. Family members might experience a child's injury like a death, but do not have this loss validated by others in the same way as a bereavement. It is the loss of the child they once knew, with some family members experiencing guilt associated with mourning despite the child's survival. Families often experience a complicated grief response associated with the injured child's recovery trajectory. Families are confronted with the complicated loss of the preinjured child and the anticipatory loss associated with the injured child's unmet or delayed milestone attainment (Collings, 2008).

Siblings experience a disruption to their sense of meaning about the safety of their world due to the unexpectedness of the ABI event and exposure to the vulnerability and powerlessness of parents. In the short term, school-aged siblings are faced with the early return to their community often ill equipped to field the attention focused on them as a result of the child's injury. In the long term, siblings can also experience grief associated with the embarrassment of their injured sibling's behavior postinjury and isolation and limitations on their own activities in the community.

The family system experiences many losses associated with the change to the family homeostasis and the resultant reorganization required for adaptation. Family Forward provides a supportive and containing environment for family members as they grapple with these losses and integrate their changed situation into their lives.

Families are typically offered trauma support and psychological first aid at the time of their child's admission to the hospital. Once the acute phase of care has ended, and the child transitions into rehabilitation, sessions focus on enabling family members to develop sensory and cognitive meanings of the trauma by putting their experience into narrative. This allows family members to present their individual experiences of the trauma and understand the different meanings each person within the family system gives to this event.

Educational materials as part of a psychoeducational process are given to parents as they begin to recognize their own trauma responses and those of their children and how they can be assisted at different ages and developmental stages. The social worker monitors the impact of the trauma on all family members in counseling sessions and refers to specialist trauma counseling services as required.

Shortly after the traumatic event that led to the child's ABI, families can interpret the term *recovery* as meaning a return to the child's preinjury function. Family perceptions of a child's injury can have implications for how the family system reorganizes itself to manage the changed needs of the injured child. It is often necessary for family members to receive and manage information about their child's injury as a gradual and paced process, allowing for the continuation of role function and coping through the rehabilitation phase (Miller, 2001). Family members' perceptions of the child's injury and recovery trajectory are monitored throughout the inpatient admission to ensure that any issues that might promote or hinder child and family recovery are identified and interventions are delivered in consultation with the family and rehabilitation team.

Family problem solving and coping

Family Forward examines family problem solving and coping by addressing family system issues related to family burden: meeting family needs and coping. Family burden is raised with families in relation to their appraisal of how the care needs of their injured child have increased and the impact this is having on the family members' health and well-being. Family Forward focuses on parents and how they are managing the increased demands of caring for the injured child in the hospital while maintaining the executive roles and responsibilities with noninjured siblings. Family Forward problem solves with parents to utilize their own finite resources to best effect while mobilizing the resources of others. Self-care plans are negotiated and formalized if agreed between the family and social worker that the burden on carers is posing a risk to adaptation.

Family Forward also monitors stress and psychological distress of family members associated with family burden. If the stress and psychological distress are assessed within normal range, then the social worker will continue to work with the family to reduce adverse effects. Referrals are made to either internal or external mental health or psychological services as required.

An integral part of intervening to reduce family members' burden, stress and psychological distress is to ensure that the family's needs postinjury are being met. Meeting family needs during the rehabilitation phase of care can be challenging during the upheaval of family systems change. Family Forward encourages families to identify their needs in relation to health information about the injured family member, emotional support, instrumental or practical support, professional support in the form of advice, community support, and familial supports that are addressed to ensure these needs are met (Kreutzer, Gervasio, & Camplair, 1994). Collaborative problem solving between the family and rehabilitation team are undertaken to ensure family needs are met in a timely manner (Patrick et al., 2012). The early identification of needs will result in families being better able to take control of the adaptation process and engage resources to support family system balance postinjury.

Family Forward facilitates discussion with families to understand the coping styles of each family member to maximize family adaptations. Family Forward assesses the preinjury and present coping strategies of all family members and how this affects the pattern of interaction in the family system. The assessment forms part of an ongoing psychosocial assessment and counseling process that engages family members in discussion about how they are coping in response to the preinjury stressors and current crisis associated with the child's injury.

Family Forward works with family members to recognize the repertoire of coping strategies used within the family system to deal with change and crisis. This process seeks to promote the positive coping strategies employed by individual family members and how these strategies interact within the whole system to achieve adaptation. Family Forward also assists families to address negative coping strategies that pose a risk to the recovery process.

Within the spousal subsystem, parents might need facilitated discussion around issues relating to differences in coping styles, the burden of caregiving, resumption of parental limit setting, parental disengagement, and marital strain. For the parent–child dyad there could be issues relating to increased responsibility placed on the noninjured siblings and distress arising from periods of separation (Waaland & Kreutzer, 1988; Wade et al., 1995; Wade et al., 1996). To optimize child and family coping during the rehabilitation phase, the social worker delivering the intervention might need to contextualize the family coping experience with the rest of the rehabilitation team (Foster & Carlson-Green, 1993) so that a collaborative approach to support family coping is in place.

Family resources

Family Forward assesses the family's informal and formal resources to assist the family adaptation process and prepare families for their community reintegration postdischarge.

Family Forward provides an ABI Family Education Pack that covers a range of material related to family experience post-ABI and resources. The resources are intended to equip families with information and knowledge that will assist them to navigate the service system during their child's reintegration into the home. The psychoeducational resources focus on the experience of other families who have a child with an ABI. The material is provided as a way of facilitating discussion with families about the needs required to support the family system as they transition home. The resources cover a range of specialist ABI services and more general services that the family can access.

Conclusion

It is important for families to have access to psychosocial interventions in the early stages of their child's ABI recovery to optimize child and family outcomes. Family Forward is a new and innovative development for social work practice targeting early recovery that is integrated into the pediatric rehabilitation service model of care. A trial is currently underway and an evaluation of Family Forward will contribute toward clinical and research knowledge in social work and rehabilitation practices in this area.

Acknowledgment

We would like to thank Kate Lawless who was helpful when we were deciding on a title for the intervention.

References

Aitken, M. E., Korehbandi, P., Parnell, D., Parker, J. G., Stefans, V., Tompkins, E., & Schulz, E. G. (2004). Experiences from the development of a comprehensive family support program for pediatric trauma and rehabilitation patients. *Archives of Physical Medicine & Rehabilitation, 86*(1), 175–179. doi:10.1016/j.apmr.2004.02.026

Anderson, V. A., Catroppa, C., Haritou, F., Morse, S., Pentland, L., Rosenfeld, J., & Stargatt, R. (2001). Predictors of acute child and family outcome following traumatic brain injury in children. *Pediatric Neurosurgery, 34*, 138–148. doi:10.1159/000056009

Australian Institute of Health & Welfare. (2007). *Disability in Australia: Acquired brain injury* (Bulletin No. 55, Cat No. AUS 96). Canberra, Australia: Author.

Benn, K. M., & McColl, M. A. (2004). Parental coping following childhood acquired brain injury. *Brain Injury, 18*, 239–255. doi:10.1080/02699050310001617343

Carnes, S. L., & Quinn, W. H. (2005). Family adaptation to brain injury: Coping and psychological distress. *Families, Systems, & Health, 23*, 186–203. doi:10.1037/1091-7527.23.2.186

Carr, A. (2012). *Family therapy: Concepts, process and practice.* Hoboken, NJ: Wiley.

Catroppa, C., Anderson, V. A., Morse, S. A., Haritou, F., & Rosenfeld, J. V. (2008). Outcome and predictors of functional recovery 5 years following pediatric traumatic brain injury (TBI). *Journal of Pediatric Psychology, 33*, 707–718. doi:10.1093/jpepsy/jsn006

Cavallo, M. M., & Kay, T. (2005). The family system. In J. M. Silver, T. W. McAllister, & S. C. Yudofsky (Eds.), *Textbook of traumatic brain injury* (pp. 533–558). Arlington, VA: American Psychiatric Publishing.

Clark, A., Stedmon, J., & Margison, S. (2008). An exploration of the experience of mothers whose children sustain traumatic brain injury (TBI) and their families. *Clinical Child Psychology & Psychiatry, 13*, 565–583. doi:10.1177/1359104508090607

Collings, C. (2008). That's not my child anymore! Parental grief after acquired brain injury (ABI): Incidence, nature and longevity. *British Journal of Social Work, 38*, 1499–1517. doi:10.1093/bjsw/bcm055

Conoley, J. C., & Sheridan, S. M. (1996). Pediatric traumatic brain injury: Challenges and interventions for families. *Journal of Learning Disabilities, 29*, 662–669. doi:10.1177/002221949602900610

Foster, M. A., & Carlson-Green, B. (1993). The transition from hospital to home: Family readjustment and response to therapeutic intervention following childhood-acquired brain injury. *Family Systems Medicine, 11*, 173–180. doi:10.1037/h0089055

Gan, C., Campbell, K. A., Gemeinhardt, M., & McFadden, G. T. (2006). Predictors of family system functioning after brain injury. *Brain Injury, 20*, 587–600. doi:10.1080/02699050600743725

Gan, C., Gargaro, J., Brandys, C., Gerber, G., & Boschen, K. (2010). Family caregivers' support needs after brain injury: A synthesis of perspectives from caregivers, programs, and researchers. *NeuroRehabilitation, 27*, 5–18.

Goldenberg, H., & Goldenberg, I. (2013). *Family therapy: An overview* (8th ed.). Belmont, CA: Brooks/Cole.

Kosciulek, J. F., McCubbin, M. A., & McCubbin, H. I. (1993). A theoretical framework for family adaptation to head injury. *Journal of Rehabilitation, 59*(3), 40–45.

Kreutzer, J. S., Gervasio, A. H., & Camplair, P. S. (1994). Primary caregivers' psychological status and family functioning after traumatic brain injury. *Brain Injury, 8*, 197–210. doi:10.3109/02699059409150973

Laroi, F. (2003). Case study: The family systems approach to treating families of persons with a brain injury: A potential collaboration between family therapist and brain injury professional. *Brain Injury, 17*, 175–187.

Lax Pericall, M. T., & Taylor, E. (2014). Family function and its relationship to injury severity and psychiatric outcome in children with acquired brain injury: A systematized review. *Developmental Medicine & Child Neurology, 56*(1), 19–30. doi:10.1111/dmcn.12237

Lezak, M. D. (1986). Psychological implications of traumatic brain damage for the patient's family. *Rehabilitation Psychology, 31,* 241–250. doi:10.1037/h0091551

Maitz, E. A., & Sachs, P. R. (1995). Treating families of individuals with traumatic brain injury from a family systems perspective. *The Journal of Head Trauma Rehabilitation, 10*(2), 1–11. doi:10.1097/00001199-199504000-00003

Martin, D. A. (1988). Children and adolescents with traumatic brain injury: Impact on the family. *Journal of Learning Disabilities, 21,* 464–470. doi:10.1177/002221948802100803

Max, J. E., Castillo, C. S., Robin, D. A., Lindgren, S. D., Smith, W. L., Jr., Sato, Y., ... Stierwalt, J. A. (1998). Predictors of family functioning after traumatic brain injury in children and adolescents. *Journal of the American Academy of Child & Adolescent Psychiatry, 37,* 83–90. doi:10.1097/00004583-199801000-00021

McCubbin, H. I., Thompson, A. I., & McCubbin, M. A. (1996). *Family assessment: Resiliency, coping and adaptation. Inventories for research and practice.* Madison, WI: University of Wisconsin.

McCubbin, M. A., McCubbin, H. I., Danielson, C. B., Hamel-Bissell, B., & Winstead-Fry, P. (1993). Families coping with illness: The resiliency model of family stress, adjustment, and adaptation. In C. Danielson, B. Hamel-Bissell, & P. Winstead-Fry (Eds.), *Families, health, and illness: Perspectives on coping and intervention* (pp. 21–61). St. Louis, MO: Mosby.

Miller, L. (2001). Family therapy of brain injury: Basic principles and innovative strategies. In M. M. MacFarlane (Ed.), *Family therapy and mental health: Innovations in theory and practice* (pp. 311–330). Binghamton, NY: Haworth Clinical Practice Press.

Patrick, P. D., Savage, R. C., Hermans, E., Winkens, I., Winkel-Witlox, S. T., & van Iperen, A. (2012). Caregiver reported problems of children and families 2–4 years following rehabilitation for pediatric brain injury. *NeuroRehabilitation, 30,* 213–217.

Perlesz, A., Furlong, M., & McLachlan, D. (1992). Family work and acquired brain injury. *Australian & New Zealand Journal of Family Therapy, 13,* 145–153.

Rivara, J. B., Fay, G. C., Jaffe, K. M., Polissar, N. L., Shurtleff, H. A., & Martin, K. M. (1992). Predictors of family functioning one year following traumatic brain injury in children. *Archives of Physical Medicine & Rehabilitation, 73,* 899–910.

Rivara, J. M. B., Jaffe, K. M., Polissar, N. L., Fay, G. C., Liao, S., & Martin, K. M. (1996). Predictors of family functioning and change 3 years after traumatic brain injury in children. *Archives of Physical Medicine & Rehabilitation, 77,* 754–764. doi:10.1016/s0003-9993(96)90253-1

Robson, T., Ziviani, J., & Spina, S. (2005). Personal experiences of families of children with a traumatic brain injury in the transition from hospital to home. *Brain Impairment, 6*(1), 45–55. doi:10.1375/brim.6.1.45.65477

Ryan, N. P., van Bijnen, L., Catroppa, C., Beauchamp, M. H., Crossley, L., Hearps, S., & Anderson, V. (2015). Longitudinal outcome and recovery of social problems after pediatric traumatic brain injury (TBI): Contribution of brain insult and family environment. *International Journal of Developmental Neuroscience, 49,* 23–30. doi:10.1016/j.ijdevneu.2015.12.004

Sambuco, M., Brookes, N., Catroppa, C., & Lah, S. (2012). Predictors of long-term sibling behavioral outcome and self-esteem following pediatric traumatic brain injury. *Journal of Head Trauma Rehabilitation, 27,* 413–423. doi:10.1097/HTR.0b013e3182274162

Schmidt, A. T., Orsten, K. D., Hanten, G. R., Li, X., & Levin, H. S. (2010). Family environment influences emotion recognition following paediatric traumatic brain injury. *Brain Injury, 24,* 1550–1560. doi:10.3109/02699052.2010.523047

Spina, S., Ziviani, J., & Nixon, J. (2005). Children, brain injury and the resiliency model of family adaptation. *Brain Impairment, 6*(1), 33–44. doi:10.1375/brim.6.1.33.65478

Stancin, T., Wade, S. L., Walz, N. C., Yeates, K. O., & Taylor, H. G. (2008). Traumatic brain injuries in early childhood: Initial impact on the family. *Journal of Developmental and Behavioral Pediatrics, 29*, 253–261. doi: 10.1097/DBP.0b013e31816b6b0f

Taylor, H., Drotar, D., Wade, S., Yeates, K., Stancin, T., & Klein, S. (1995). Recovery from TBI in children: The importance of the family. In M. E. Michel (Ed.), *Traumatic head injury in children* (pp. 188–216). New York, NY: Oxford University Press.

Waaland, P. K., & Kreutzer, J. S. (1988). Family response to childhood traumatic brain injury. *Journal of Head Trauma Rehabilitation, 3*(4), 51–63. doi:10.1097/00001199-198812000-00008

Wade, S. L., Borawski, E. A., Taylor, H. G., Drotar, D., Yeates, K. O., & Stancin, T. (2001). The relationship of caregiver coping to family outcomes during the initial year following pediatric traumatic injury. *Journal of Consulting and Clinical Psychology, 69*, 406–415. doi:10.1037/0022-006x.69.3.406

Wade, S., Drotar, D., Taylor, H. G., & Stancin, T. (1995). Assessing the effects of traumatic brain injury on family functioning: Conceptual and methodological issues. *Journal of Pediatric Psychology, 20*, 737–752. doi:10.1093/jpepsy/20.6.737

Wade, S. L., Michaud, L., & Brown, T. M. (2006). Putting the pieces together: Preliminary efficacy of a family problem-solving intervention for children with traumatic brain injury. *Journal of Head Trauma Rehabilitation, 21*(1), 57–67. doi:10.1097/00001199-200601000-00006

Wade, S. L., Taylor, G., Drotar, D., Stancin, T., Yeates, K. O., & Minich, N. M. (2003). Parent–adolescent interactions after traumatic brain injury. *Journal of Head Trauma Rehabilitation, 18*(2), 164–176. doi:10.1097/00001199-200303000-00007

Wade, S. L., Taylor, H. G., Drotar, D., Stancin, T., & Yeates, K. O. (1996). Childhood traumatic brain injury: Initial impact on the family. *Journal of Learning Disabilities, 29*, 652–661. doi:10.1177/002221949602900609

Wade, S. L., Taylor, H. G., Drotar, D., Stancin, T., & Yeates, K. O. (1998). Family burden and adaptation during the initial year after traumatic brain injury in children. *Pediatrics, 102*(1), 110–116. doi:10.1542/peds.102.1.110

Wade, S. L., Taylor, H. G., Drotar, D., Stancin, T., Yeates, K. O., & Minich, N. M. (2002). A prospective study of long-term caregiver and family adaptation following brain injury in children. *Journal of Head Trauma Rehabilitation, 17*(2), 96–111. doi:10.1097/00001199-200204000-00003

Wade, S. L., Taylor, H. G., Yeates, K. O., Drotar, D., Stancin, T., Minich, N. M., & Schluchter, M. (2006). Long-term parental and family adaptation following pediatric brain injury. *Journal of Pediatric Psychology, 31*, 1072–1083. doi:10.1093/jpepsy/jsj077

Wade, S. L., Walz, N. C., Cassedy, A., Taylor, H. G., Stancin, T., & Yeates, K. O. (2010). Caregiver functioning following early childhood TBI: Do moms and dads respond differently? *NeuroRehabilitation, 27*(1), 63–72.

Yeates, K. O., Taylor, H. G., Walz, N. C., Stancin, T., & Wade, S. L. (2010). The family environment as a moderator of psychosocial outcomes following traumatic brain injury in young children. *Neuropsychology, 24*, 345–356. doi:10.1037/a0018387

Ylvisaker, M., Adelson, D., Braga, L. W., Burnett, S. M., Glang, A., Feeney, T., … Todis, B. (2005). Rehabilitation and ongoing support after pediatric TBI. *Journal of Head Trauma Rehabilitation, 20*(1), 95–109. doi:10.1097/00001199-200501000-00009

Zittel, K. M., Lawrence, S., & Wodarski, J. S. (2002). Biopsychosocial model of health and healing: Implications for health social work practice. *Journal of Human Behavior in the Social Environment, 5*(1), 19–33. doi:10.1300/j137v05n01_02

Self-Advocacy for Independent Life: A Program for Personal Self Advocacy after Brain Injury

Lenore A. Hawley

ABSTRACT

Traumatic brain injury (TBI) can result in long-term injury-related disabilities. Individuals with TBI and their families must often advocate for themselves to secure resources to address their postinjury needs. However, the ability to advocate may be compromised by the effects of the injury. The Self-Advocacy for Independent Life (SAIL) program aims to empower individuals and families with the skills of self-advocacy so they can navigate life after brain injury in a self-efficacious manner.

An estimated 1.7 million Americans sustain traumatic brain injury (TBI) each year (Faul, Wald, & Coronado, 2010). Many recover from these injuries, but an estimated 124,626 Americans annually are left with long-term TBI-related disabilities (Selassie et al., 2008). TBI can lead to changes in many aspects of an individual's life, affecting physical, emotional, social, vocational, and financial functioning (Johnstone, Mount, & Schopp, 2003; Levin, Grossman, Rose, & Teasdale, 1979; Morton & Wehman, 1995; Rao & Lyketsos, 2000). Individuals who have sustained TBI often need services and resources not required prior to the injury (Heinemann, Sokol, Garvin, & Bode, 2002). These services include rehabilitation therapies, psychosocial counseling and support, specialized medical services, vocational rehabilitation, transportation assistance, financial support, and family services.

Appropriate resources may be difficult to find and access (Pickelsimer et al., 2007). Approximately 40% of individuals hospitalized with TBI report at least one unmet need for services a year after TBI (Corrigan, Whiteneck, & Mellick, 2004). Individuals and families often receive only minimal information regarding the long-term challenges of life following TBI (Hibbard et al., 2002). Accessing these resources may require the individual or a family member to engage in self-advocacy. Despite this need for self-advocacy, little has been done to provide evidence-based programs to develop advocacy skills for individuals with TBI and their families. This article defines self-advocacy, describes the need for self-advocacy training following TBI, reviews some of the relevant self-advocacy research, and describes an intervention designed to empower individuals with TBI and families with the skills of self-advocacy.

Self-advocacy after TBI

Advocacy is defined as supporting or recommending a particular cause or policy (Oxford Dictionary Online, n.d.). Several types of advocacy have been described in the literature, including peer advocacy (advocating for others who are facing similar challenges), systems advocacy (advocating to change policy, laws, or rules for a specific cause), and self-advocacy (Advocacy, n.d.). Self-advocacy is a concept that has been promoted for numerous groups who are in need of health and social services, including people with disabilities (Hagan & Donovan, 2013). Self-advocacy has been defined as asserting your own needs and taking action to fulfill those needs (Hawley, 1992, 2008, 2014). It involves tasks such as assessing one's own needs, gathering resources, problem solving, communicating, and negotiating to get needs met (Hawley, 1992, 2008, 2014; Roberts, Ju, & Zhang, 2016; Test, Fowler, Wood, Brewer, & Eddy, 2005). Although the need for self-advocacy increases after TBI, the injured individual's ability to self-advocate could be compromised by the cognitive, communicative, and emotional effects of the injury (Ylvisaker & Feeney, 1996). The injured individual may have self-advocated prior to the injury (e.g., when solving a conflict with a landlord, or applying for a new job). However, his or her ability to communicate needs, problem solve situations, remember details, and complete tasks may now be impaired.

A family member could also take on the role of self-advocate, advocating along with or in place of the injured person, depending on the severity of the disability (e.g., when the injured individual is unable to communicate, or unable to retain information day to day). In this role, the family member could advocate for the needs of the injured person, but might also be advocating for his or her own needs as a caregiver and for the needs of the family as a whole. Families of individuals with TBI often need financial support, educational information, respite care, psychological support, and other resources (Degeneffe, 2001; Degeneffe, Chang, Dunlap, Man, & Sung, 2011; Man, 1998; Tverdov, McClure, Brownsberger, & Armstrong, 2016). Families report that appropriate services and resources are limited (Tverdov et al., 2016). The need for advocacy following TBI occurs at a time when the family is facing an increased burden and stress due to the effects of the injury (Hall et al., 1994; Verhaeghe, Defloor, & Grypdonck, 2005). Thus, self-advocacy following TBI can be challenging for both the injured individual and for the family members who advocate for or with the individual. The combination of unmet needs, limited resources, and injury-related challenges points to a pressing need for self-advocacy support and training for individuals with TBI and families.

Self-advocacy in other populations

Self-advocacy programs have been developed to address the needs of other populations. Programs have been described for children and adults with various disabilities (e.g., developmental disabilities, learning disabilities, mental illness), for parents and families of individuals with disabilities, and for individuals with specific health conditions such as cancer or kidney disease (Curtin et al., 2008; Dawson, n.d.; Hagan & Medberry, 2015; Kissel, 2006; Test et al., 2005). These interventions often focus on addressing the beliefs, knowledge, and behaviors needed to personally advocate for oneself or family. Many of these interventions emphasize increasing awareness of one's own needs, gaining knowledge of resources, and developing effective communication skills (Hagan & Medberry, 2015; Kissel, 2006; Merchant & Gajar, 1997; Test et al., 2005). In addition, some self-advocacy programs also address systems advocacy, advocating for changes in policies and laws that affect the disability or health condition with which the individual is aligned (Test et al., 2005).

Self-advocacy research related to TBI

Ylvisaker and Feeney (1996) pointed out the need for self-advocacy support and training for individuals with TBI, and outlined the difficulties facing this population, as they strive to advocate for themselves. However, research regarding self-advocacy interventions for individuals with TBI is scarce. A few studies have been published, most emphasizing family advocacy. Man (1998) developed a Family Empowerment Questionnaire, based on a sample of 211 family members of individuals with acquired brain injury. His research suggested that efficacy beliefs appear to be the most important factor in a family member's ability to cope with the challenges of life after brain injury (Man, 1998). He later investigated an intervention program for family members, which was found to improve family empowerment (Man, 1999). Glang, McLaughlin, and Schroeder (2007) demonstrated the efficacy of an advocacy communication skills program for parents of children with TBI. More recently, Brown et al. (2015) investigated a self-advocacy intervention for people with TBI and family members, which provided an overview of TBI and advocacy with an emphasis on policymaking and community organizing. They found that a curriculum-based program addressing community advocacy was not superior to a self-directed program, and concluded that it was beneficial to gather like-minded people together to discuss advocacy (Brown et al., 2015).

Recently, TBI has been increasingly described as a chronic disease, stressing the lifelong consequences of the injury (Masel, 2009). Evidence-based self-advocacy interventions are needed to enhance the beliefs, skills, and behaviors required for individuals and families to advocate for their own needs following TBI, so that they can successfully address the long-term challenges of life after TBI.

The self-advocacy for independent life program

The Self-Advocacy for Independent Life (SAIL) program was developed through the Brain Injury Alliance of Colorado (BIAC), formerly the Brain Injury Association of Colorado. The program was developed to empower individuals with brain injury and their family members with the skills of personal self-advocacy. A committee was formed through BIAC, composed of consumers and professionals, with the goal of developing a self-advocacy program for family members of individuals with TBI. The author led the development of the program. After completing a needs assessment and review of the literature, it was determined that such a program should address self-advocacy for both family members and individuals with TBI. Working in collaboration with a subcommittee of consumers and rehabilitation professionals, the SAIL program was designed to increase self-advocacy beliefs, knowledge and behaviors. The program involved interactive self-advocacy workshops along with a workbook.

Single-day SAIL workshops were completed in numerous locations throughout the state of Colorado, directed toward both individuals with brain injury who advocate for themselves and family members who assist in advocacy efforts. These preliminary workshops were 4 hr in length, with 15 to 25 participants per workshop including both individuals with TBI and families, and followed an interactive educational group format. Anecdotal feedback and satisfaction questionnaires indicated the program was well received. Participants requested further workshops covering additional advocacy topics and time for practice of skills. A preliminary multiday workshop was held with an expanded curriculum. Participants were seven individuals with TBI, ranging from 2 to 25 years postinjury, with moderate to severe injuries. Participant feedback was positive, with comments such as "This has changed my life." Several participants reported that, because of the program, they had visited each other's homes to help each other develop organizational tools and strategies. Participants set individual goals that were scaled using Goal Attainment Scaling (GAS) (Kiresuk, Smith, & Cardillo, 1994). All participants met their individual goals. Goals included developing a personal organization system, finding transportation resources in the community, and making assertive comments during conversations with family.

Theoretical basis of the SAIL model

As mentioned, many self-advocacy programs aim to develop the beliefs, knowledge, and behaviors for successful self-advocacy. An individual's *belief* in his or her ability to succeed at a specific task is referred to as self-efficacy (Bandura, 1977). Perceived self-efficacy is strongly associated with life satisfaction and life quality post-TBI, and it has been recommended that TBI treatment should address self-efficacy (Brands, Kohler, Stapert, Wade, & van Heugten, 2014; Cicerone & Azulay, 2007). Increased self-efficacy has also been described as a targeted outcome for brain injury rehabilitation research (Man, Soong, Tam, & Hui-Chan, 2006). Enhancing self-efficacy beliefs is an important focus of the SAIL program, and the concept of self-efficacy provides a theoretical cornerstone for the program (Bandura, 1977).

The concept of self-efficacy is a component of social learning theory (Bandura, 1971), a commonly used theory in social work practice (Thyer & Myers, 2011). Social learning theory is based on the idea that individuals learn through observation, modeling, and social reinforcement. Bandura (1971) described four factors to consider in developing self-efficacy expectations: performance accomplishment or mastery of a skill, vicarious experiences or modeling, verbal persuasion, and emotional arousal. Performance accomplishment or mastery occurs through modeling and exposure to tasks and behaviors; vicarious experience is enhanced through modeling of behaviors; verbal persuasion can consist of suggestion, encouragement, and instruction; and emotional arousal can be regulated through relaxation, feedback, and exposure to ideas and events in a supportive environment (Bandura, 1977). These four self-efficacy constructs are integrated into the interactive workshop model used in SAIL. Workshop participants set individual goals regarding self-advocacy and receive feedback from others in the group regarding progress on those goals, reinforcing behavioral progress and accomplishments. Participants give and receive feedback and reinforcement from others, model and observe successful behaviors and skills, problem solve real-life self-advocacy situations, and provide each other with emotional support and encouragement. Strategies for emotional regulation and stress reduction are discussed.

The SAIL process also draws on Yalom's theory of group psychotherapy emphasizing therapeutic factors of group process (Yalom & Leszcz, 2005). One of these therapeutic factors is universality, the realization that one is not alone in addressing challenges. Individuals and families facing a disability or stressor in life may feel alone and unique in the challenges they face. Bringing people together to discuss common needs can lead to a sense of relief and normalization, and the realization that one is not unique and that others have found successes in self-advocacy (Klonoff, 2010).

Content of the SAIL program

SAIL workshops were developed specifically to address the self-advocacy needs of individuals with brain injury and their families. The content includes information on understanding brain injury and increasing knowledge of resources specific to the needs of this population. Sessions include breaks to account for cognitive fatigue. The content and process of the sessions is designed to address the cognitive needs of this population. Information from previous weeks is reviewed each week, and is provided in a written format to facilitate recall of information. The content covered in the SAIL workshops also draws on the construct of self-efficacy. SAIL emphasizes four key elements: (a) taking care of oneself in preparation for the job of self-advocacy; (b) gathering information and resources; (c) developing organizational skills; and (d) assertively communicating and negotiating (Hawley, 1992, 2008, 2014).

Take care of yourself

A TBI can disrupt routines and activities for the individual and family. Routines such as regular exercise, healthy meals, relaxation, and getting a good night's sleep might be pushed aside as the family takes on the daily challenges of life after TBI. The role of self-advocacy requires energy, clear thinking, good interpersonal skills, and emotional regulation. Within the SAIL program, a self-advocate's first task is to take care of himself or herself to advocate successfully. Family members, who have been focused on the needs of the injured person, may especially need to be reminded that taking care of oneself is a necessity rather than a luxury. The injured individual could be experiencing cognitive and physical fatigue, pain, stress and other symptoms that can interfere with self-advocacy efforts. SAIL participants learn and discuss strategies for physical and emotional self-care.

Gather information and resources

The individual with TBI needs information and resources regarding a variety of areas, such as ongoing therapy, transportation, financial assistance, psychosocial support, and legal assistance (Heinemann et al., 2002). Being informed includes being knowledgeable about the injury so that one can describe the need, know what resources are available, and know one's rights. Being informed and knowledgeable allows one to feel a sense of mastery and accomplishment. The SAIL program provides (a) basic information and ter-minology about TBI, and (b) information regarding community resources in the areas of rehabilitation, consumer advocacy, vocational reentry, trans-portation, recreation, and disability rights. Guest speakers from community agencies are invited into the group to share resources and answer questions. In addition, group members are encouraged to share information and resources with each other.

Develop organizational skills

Particularly for the individual with TBI, being organized and prepared when approaching self-advocacy can be a challenging task (Ylvisaker & Feeney, 1996). The individual and family might learn to assess their needs and gather information about resources, but could be overwhelmed by the enormity of the need and the variety and complexity of community resources. Applying for resources can be a cumbersome and confusing process. When one is organized and prepared for a phone call or a meeting, others might pay more attention and feel more accountable. The SAIL program provides strategies for organizing information, documenting conversations so that one can substantiate what has occurred, and arrive at appointments prepared and ready. Participants problem solve potential potholes, discuss strategies, and encourage each other's efforts. This focus on organization and preparation aims to reduce emotional stress and increase the belief in one's ability to master the tasks at hand.

Assertively communicate and negotiate

Most self-advocacy tasks involve communication. Self-advocacy activities include phone calls, meetings, and written communications. For the person with TBI, interpersonal communication skills can be difficult (Dahlberg et al., 2007; McDonald et al., 2008). The effects of the injury may impair a person's word finding, turn-taking, listening skills, respecting of boundaries, and emotional regulation. For both the injured person and the family member, the stress of the injury could make it difficult to communicate needs assertively. The SAIL program discusses the skill of communication in a clear, assertive manner, rather than passively or aggressively. *Assertive communication* is defined as attacking the problem, not the person, and speaking in a manner that is straightforward and respectful of the other person (Alberti & Emmons, 1990). The group practices and problem solves strategies for assertive interactions and negotiations in a variety of situations. This provides the opportunity for vicarious learning, reducing emotional stress and increasing mastery of communication skills.

Inclusion criteria and composition

SAIL workshops can include people with TBI who are advocating for themselves, family members who are advocating for or with a person with TBI, or a combination of both of these groups. Multifamily interventions that include both families and individuals with TBI have been shown to have positive effects and to be well-accepted by participants (Straits-Troster et al., 2013; Backhaus, Ibarra, Parrott, & Malec, 2016). Workshops are aimed toward individuals and families who face multiple ongoing challenges post-TBI, and have a need to self-advocate to address those needs.

Participants appear best suited for the group after intensive rehabilitation has been completed, usually 6 months or more postinjury. This allows time to develop an awareness of the need for self-advocacy as the individual returns to the community and begins to face challenges related to the injury (e.g., difficulty returning to work, obstacles in gaining financial resources, transportation issues, etc.). For individuals with TBI, additional criteria for participation include (a) being age 18 or older, (b) the ability to sustain attention in a group setting over several hours, with intermittent breaks, and (c) being responsible for conducting at least some self-management and self-advocacy tasks (e.g., making appointments, searching for resources, initiating phone conversations with resource providers).

The size of the workshop is determined in part by who is in the group. Workshops for individuals with TBI have been successful with 8 to 10 group members, allowing all participants the chance to ask questions and practice strategies. Workshops for family members have been completed with 16 to 25 participants. Groups with combined participants have also been conducted. Such combined workshops are particularly useful in rural areas, where there are smaller numbers of individuals in need. These appear to work best with 10 to 15 participants, using smaller break-out sessions within the workshop for both family members and individuals with TBI. Break-out sessions allow group members to practice skills and discuss experiences with peers in a more intimate setting.

SAIL workshops are structured in a series of four to six sessions (see Figure 1). Sessions are approximately 3 hr in length with breaks provided. Sessions are held once a week on concurrent weeks, with the exception of the last session, which takes place a month later. This provides an opportunity for participants to practice skills and problem solve situations in their lives, and then return to the final session for feedback and group problem solving.

Research regarding the SAIL intervention

The Craig Hospital Foundation recently funded a research study investigating the feasibility of the SAIL intervention for improving self-efficacy, satisfaction with life, and self-advocacy behaviors. This was a pilot feasibility study with participants randomized to either a treatment group (receiving four-session workshops and a workbook) or a control group (receiving the workbook only). Twelve individuals who sustained brain injury were enrolled in this study. Participants were required to be 18 years of age or older, English speaking, having completed inpatient rehabilitation, and at least 6 months postinjury. Self-report measures of self-efficacy and satisfaction with life were used, as well as a novel measure of self-advocacy behavior. The methodology and intervention were

Session 1
9:00: Introductions
9:15: Self Advocacy after BI – what is it
10:00: Break
10:10: Understanding BI – what do I need to know
11:00: Break
11:10: Self-assessment – what are my strengths and obstacles
11:20: Setting my own self advocacy goals
11:45: Home assignment

Session 2
9:00: Reintroductions; review of Session 1
9:15: Home assignment: review of Self-assessment
9:45: Finalizing SA goals
10:00: Break
10:15: Assertively Communicating my Needs
11:00: Break
11:15: Review and Discussion
11:45: Home assignment

Session 3
9:00: Reintroductions and review
9:30: Progress on your goals
9:45: Taking care of yourself
10:30: Break
10:45: Getting Organized
11:15: Practice and problem solving
11:45: Homework

Session 4
9:00: Reintroductions and review
9:30: Progress on goals
10:00: Problem solving
10:30: Break
10:45: Maintaining knowledge, skills, and beliefs
11:15: Developing an Action Plan
11:45: Group closure

Figure 1. Intervention workshop outline.

shown to be feasible, indicating appropriateness for further research. A more detailed description of this study has been submitted for publication.

Conclusions

The complex sequelae of TBI often lead to the need for self-advocacy on the part of the individual with the injury, a family member, or both. Being a successful self-advocate after TBI can be challenging for both the individual with TBI and family members who are involved in the process. Individuals and families could benefit from a program designed to empower them with the self-efficacy, information, and behaviors for successful self-advocacy. The SAIL program offers a model for self-advocacy intervention, addressing self-efficacy beliefs and behaviors in a structured group format. Initial pilot study data have been collected and demonstrate the feasibility of further study of this intervention for individuals with TBI. A randomized controlled trial is needed to test the efficacy of this intervention. Such a trial should target individuals who have completed inpatient rehabilitation and who are facing continued TBI challenges in the community. Further study of the replication of this intervention in various settings is also warranted. In addition, the feasibility of this intervention for family members as self-advocates should be tested.

Funding

The development of the SAIL intervention was originally funded through a grant from the Rocky Mountain Regional Brain Injury Center. Subsequent funding came from the Colorado Developmental Disabilities Planning Council, the Colorado Department of Health, and the Colorado Traumatic Brain Injury Trust Fund. Pilot research was funded through the Craig Hospital Foundation.

References

Advocacy. (n.d.). West Virginia University, Center for Excellence in Disabilities. Retrieved from http://cedwvu.org/advocacy/types-of-advocacy.php

Alberti, R., & Emmons, M. (1990). *Your perfect right: A guide to assertive living.* San Luis Obispo, CA: Impact.

Backhaus, S., Ibarra, S., Parrott, D., & Malec, J. (2016). Comparison of a cognitive-behavioral coping skills group to a peer support group in a brain injury population. *Archives in Physical Medicine and Rehabilitation, 97,* 281–291. doi:10.1016/j.apmr.2015.10.097

Bandura, A. (1971). *Social learning theory.* New York, NY: General Learning Press.

Bandura, A. (1977). Self-efficacy: Toward a unifying theory of behavioral change. *Psychological Review, 84,* 191–215. doi:10.1037/0033-295x.84.2.191

Brands, I., Kohler, S., Stapert, S., Wade, D., & van Heugten, C. (2014). Influence of self-efficacy and coping on quality of life and social participation after acquired brain injury: A 1-year follow-up study. *Archives of Physical Medicine and Rehabilitation, 95,* 2327–2334. doi:10.1016/j.apmr.2014.06.006

Brown, A. W., Moessner, A. M., Bergquist, T. F., Kendall, K. S., Diehl, N. N., & Mandrekar, J. (2015). A randomized practical behavioural trial of curriculum-based advocacy training for individuals with traumatic brain injury and their families. *Brain Injury, 29,* 1530–1538. doi:10.3109/02699052.2015.1075173

Cicerone, K., & Azulay, J. (2007). Perceived self-efficacy and life satisfaction after traumatic brain injury. *Journal of Head Trauma Rehabilitation, 22,* 257–266. doi:10.1097/01.htr.0000290970.56130.81

Corrigan, J., Whiteneck, G., & Mellick, D. (2004). Perceived needs following traumatic brain injury. *Journal of Head Trauma Rehabilitation, 19,* 205–216.

Curtin, R. B., Walters, B. A., Schatell, D., Pennell, P., Wise, M., & Klicko, K. (2008). Self-efficacy and self-management behaviors in patients with chronic kidney disease. *Advances in Chronic Kidney Disease, 15,* 191–205. doi:10.1053/j.ackd.2008.01.006

Dahlberg, C. A., Cusick, C. P., Hawley, L. A., Newman, J. K., Morey, C. E., Harrison-Felix, C. L., & Whiteneck, G. G. (2007). Treatment efficacy of social communication skills training after traumatic brain injury: A randomized treatment and deferred treatment controlled trial. *Archives in Physical Medicine and Rehabilitation, 88,* 1561–1573. doi:10.1016/j.apmr.2007.07.033

Dawson, J. (n.d.). Self advocacy: A valuable skill for your teenager with LD. *LD Online.* Retrieved from http://www.ldonline.org/article/Self-Advocacy

Degeneffe, C. E. (2001). Family caregiving and traumatic brain injury. *Health Social Work, 26,* 257–268. doi:10.1093/hsw/26.4.257

Degeneffe, C. E., Chang, F., Dunlap, L., Man, D., & Sung, C. (2011). Development and validation of the caregiver empowerment scale: A resource for working with family caregivers of persons with traumatic brain injury. *Rehabilitation Psychology, 56,* 243–250. doi:10.1037/a0024465

Faul, M. X. L., Wald, M. M., & Coronado, V. G. (2010). *Traumatic brain injury in the United States: Emergency department visits, hospitalizations, and deaths.* Retrieved from www.cdc. gov/traumaticbraininjury

Glang, A., McLaughlin, K., & Schroeder, S. (2007). Using interactive multimedia to teach parent advocacy skills: An exploratory study. *Journal of Head Trauma Rehabilitation, 22,* 198–205. doi:10.1097/01.HTR.0000271121.42523.3a00001199-200705000-00007[pii]

Hagan, T. L., & Donovan, H. S. (2013). Self-advocacy and cancer: A concept analysis. *Journal of Advanced Nursing, 69,* 2348–2359. doi:10.1111/jan.12084

Hagan, T. L., & Medberry, E. (2015). Patient education vs. patient experiences of self-advocacy: Changing the discourse to support cancer survivors. *Journal of Cancer Education, 31,* 375–381. doi:10.1007/s13187-015-0828-x

Hall, K. M., Karzmark, P., Stevens, M., Englander, J., O'Hare, P., & Wright, J. (1994). Family stressors in traumatic brain injury: A two-year follow-up. *Archives in Physical Medicine and Rehabilitation, 75,* 876–884. doi:10.1016/0003-9993(94)90112-0

Hawley, L. (1992, 2008, 2014). Self advocacy after brain injury. In L. Hawley (Ed.), *SAIL: Self advocacy for independent life,* (pp. 11–27). Denver, CO: Brain Injury Association of Colorado.

Heinemann, A. W., Sokol, K., Garvin, L., & Bode, R. K. (2002). Measuring unmet needs and services among persons with traumatic brain injury. *Archives in Physical Medicine and Rehabilitation, 83,* 1052–1059.

Hibbard, M. R., Cantor, J., Charatz, H., Rosenthal, R., Ashman, T., Gundersen, N., … Gartner, A. (2002). Peer support in the community: Initial findings of a mentoring program for individuals with traumatic brain injury and their families. *Journal of Head Trauma Rehabilitation, 17,* 112–131. doi:10.1097/00001199-200204000-00004

Johnstone, B., Mount, D., & Schopp, L. H. (2003). Financial and vocational outcomes 1 year after traumatic brain injury. *Archives in Physical Medicine and Rehabilitation, 84,* 238–241. doi:10.1053/apmr.2003.50097

Kiresuk, T. J., Smith, A., & Cardillo, J. E. (Eds.). (1994). *Goal attainment scaling: Applications, theory, and measurement.* Hillsdale, NJ: Erlbaum.

Kissel, H. (2006, April). *Self-advocacy programs for college students with disabilities: A framework for assessment.* Paper presented at the American Educational Research Association Annual Conference, San Francisco, CA.

Klonoff, P. (2010). *Psychotherpay after brain injury: Principles and techniques.* New York, NY: Guilford.

Levin, H. S., Grossman, R. G., Rose, J. E., & Teasdale, G. (1979). Long-term neuropsychological outcome of closed head injury. *Journal of Neurosurgery, 50,* 412–422. doi:10.3171/ jns.1979.50.4.0412

Man, D. (1998). The empowering of Hong Kong Chinese families with a brain damaged member: Its investigation and measurement. *Brain Injury, 12*, 245–254. doi:10.1080/026990598122728

Man, D. (1999). Community-based empowerment programme for families with a brain injured survivor: An outcome study. *Brain Injury, 13*, 433–445. doi:10.1080/026990599121485

Man, D., Soong, W., Tam, S., & Hui-Chan, C. (2006). Self-efficacy outcomes of people with brain injury in cognitive skill training using different types of trainer-trainee interaction. *Brain Injury, 20*, 959–970. doi:10.1080/02699050600909789

Masel, B. (2009). *Conceptualizing brain injury as a chronic disease.* Vienna, VA: The Brain Injury Association of America.

McDonald, S., Tate, R., Togher, L., Bornhofen, C., Long, E., Gertler, P., & Bowen, R. (2008). Social skills treatment for people with severe, chronic acquired brain injuries: A multicenter trial. *Archives in Physical Medicine and Rehabilitation, 89*, 1648–1659. doi:10.1016/j.apmr.2008.02.029

Merchant, D., & Gajar, A. (1997). A review of the literature on self advocacy components in transition programs for students with learning disabilities. *Journal of Vocational Rehabilitation, 8*, 223–231.

Morton, M. V., & Wehman, P. (1995). Psychosocial and emotional sequelae of individuals with traumatic brain injury: A literature review and recommendations. *Brain Injury, 9*, 81–92. doi:10.3109/02699059509004574

Oxford Dictionary Online. (n.d.). Retrieved from http://www.oxforddictionaries.com/us/definition/american_english/advocacy

Pickelsimer, E. E., Selassie, A. W., Sample, P. L., Heinemann, A. W., Gu, J. K., & Veldheer, L. C. (2007). Unmet service needs of persons with traumatic brain injury. *Journal of Head Trauma Rehabilitation, 22*(1), 1–13. doi:10.1097/00001199-200701000-00001

Rao, V., & Lyketsos, C. (2000). Neuropsychiatric sequelae of traumatic brain injury. *Psychosomatics, 41*(2), 95–103. doi:10.1176/appi.psy.41.2.95

Roberts, E., Ju, S., & Zhang, D. (2016). Review of practices that promote self-advocacy for students with disabilities. *Journal of Disability Policy Studies, 26*, 209–220. doi:10.1177/1044207314540213

Selassie, A. W., Zaloshnja, E., Langlois, J. A., Miller, T., Jones, P., & Steiner, C. (2008). Incidence of long-term disability following traumatic brain injury hospitalization, United States, 2003. *Journal of Head Trauma Rehabilitation, 23*, 123–131. doi:10.1097/01.HTR.0000314531.30401.39

Straits-Troster, K., Gierisch, J. M., Strauss, J. L., Dyck, D. G., Dixon, L. B., Norell, D., & Perlick, D. A. (2013). Multifamily group treatment for veterans with traumatic brain injury: What is the value to participants? *Psychiatric Services, 64*, 541–546. doi:10.1176/appi.ps.001632012

Test, D., Fowler, C., Wood, W., Brewer, D., & Eddy, S. (2005). A conceptual framework of self-advocacy for students with disabilities. *Remedial and Special Education, 26*(1), 41–54. doi:10.1177/07419325050260010601

Thyer, B., & Myers, L. (2011). Behavioral and cognitive theories. In J. Brandell (Ed.), *Theory and practice in clinical social work*, (pp. 21–40). Los Angeles, CA: Sage.

Tverdov, A. H., McClure, K. S., Brownsberger, M. G., & Armstrong, S. L. (2016). Family needs at a post-acute rehabilitation setting and suggestions for supports. *Brain Injury, 30*, 324–333. doi:10.3109/02699052.2015.1113566

Verhaeghe, S., Defloor, T., & Grypdonck, M. (2005). Stress and coping among families of patients with traumatic brain injury: A review of the literature. *Journal of Clinical Nursing, 14*, 1004–1012. doi:10.1111/j.1365-2702.2005.01126.x

Yalom, I., & Leszcz, M. (2005). *The theory and practice of group psychotherapy* (5th ed.) New York, NY: Basic Books.

Ylvisaker, M., & Feeney, T. J. (1996). Executive functions after traumatic brain injury: Supported cognition and self-advocacy. *Seminars in Speech and Language, 17*, 217–232. doi:10.1055/s-2008-1064100

Describing an Early Social Work Intervention Program for Families after Severe Traumatic Brain Injury

Grahame Simpson, Daniella Pfeiffer, Shay Keogh, and Brigitte Lane

ABSTRACT

A necessary step to evaluating practice is the accurate specification of social work interventions. Interventions delivered to 27 families with a relative with traumatic brain injury (TBI) admitted to a specialist inpatient brain injury rehabilitation service were coded (655 hr of social work services). The most frequent interventions were counseling, education, and case management. Services addressed person-oriented (65%; e.g., adjustment to hospital, adjustment to disability, family conflict) and environment-oriented (35%; e.g., transport, accommodation, finance, legal, and immigration) issues. This is the first description of a family intervention program after TBI delivered in an inpatient setting and lays the groundwork for future evaluation.

Traumatic brain injury (TBI) is a global public health issue (Frost, Farrer, Primosch, & Hedges, 2013). In the United States alone, 1.5 to 2 million people are estimated to sustain a TBI every year (Langlois, Rutland-Brown, & Wald, 2006). In Australia, the annual incidence of TBI resulting in hospitalizations is estimated to be 100 per 100,000 (Tate, McDonald, & Lulham, 1998) and costs the Australian economy $8.6 billion per year (Access Economics, 2008). Across Western developed countries, the common causes of TBI sustained by civilians are road accidents, falls, assaults, sporting injuries, and gunshot wounds (Langlois et al., 2006; Peeters et al., 2015; Tate et al., 1998). TBIs are also common in conflict zones and TBI has been described as the "signature injury" of the wars in Afghanistan and Iraq (Warden, 2006). A TBI is classified as severe (in contrast to a mild or moderate injury) if post traumatic amnesia (PTA) lasts for longer than 24 hr (Russell & Smith, 1961; Teasdale, 1995).

The common consequences of severe TBI span motor-sensory, cognitive, communication, and behavioral domains (Baker, Tandy, & Dixon, 2002; Degeneffe, 2001; Simpson, Simons, & McFadyen, 2002). People with severe

TBI commonly report problems with attention, speed of information processing, memory, executive functions, anger control, and broader disinhibited or impulsive behaviors (Daisley, Tams, & Kischka, 2009). The continuum of recovery after severe TBI typically involves initial acute medical care, followed by inpatient rehabilitation and then longer term community-based rehabilitation (Carlton & Stephenson, 1990; Khan, Baguley, & Cameron, 2003; Simpson et al., 2002; Tverdov, McClure, Brownsberger, & Armstrong, 2016). Although a proportion of people make a full recovery after severe TBI, the majority will experience ongoing challenges in activity and participation in areas such as occupation, relationships, and independent living (Baker et al., 2002; Simpson et al., 2002).

The effects on family members when a relative sustains severe TBI can be widespread and multilayered (Degeneffe, 2001; Sander, Maestas, Clark, & Havins, 2013; Winstanley, Simpson, Tate, & Miles, 2006), with brain damage characterized as a "family affair" (Lezak, 1988). All members of the family system can be affected (Degeneffe & Olney, 2008; Perlesz, Kinsella, & Crowe, 2000). Depression or anxiety is common among family members, with rates between 20% and 40% (Anderson, Simpson, & Morey, 2013; Anderson et al., 2009; Kreutzer et al., 2009). Anxiety in particular has been reported as early as 3 to 6 months postinjury (Livingston, Brooks, & Bond, 1985; Marsh, Kersel, Havill, & Sleigh, 1998). The impact on family functioning can include reduced affective involvement, communication, general functioning, and role change (Anderson et al., 2013; Anderson et al., 2009; Kreutzer et al., 2009). Instrumental impacts can include reduced family income, reduced hours of work, and higher levels of help-seeking behavior and medication use (Hall et al., 1994).

This project focused on the social work interventions delivered during the inpatient rehabilitation phase at the Liverpool Brain Injury Rehabilitation Unit (LBIRU) at Liverpool Hospital, Sydney, Australia. Within the Australian context, social workers intervene with both clients with TBI and their families during this phase (Simpson et al., 2002). However, to the best of our knowledge, there have been no evaluations of the efficacy of social work interventions, reflecting the limited evaluation of social work services within health settings more generally (Judd & Sheffield, 2010).

As the first step toward evaluation, a number of authors have emphasized the importance of being able to accurately specify the nature of the social work interventions that are delivered (Chambless & Hollon, 1998; Rosen, Proctor, & Staudt, 1999; Royse, 2008). Therefore, to help maximize specificity, this study targeted the interventions provided to families (rather than families and clients) for three reasons. First, in Australia, social workers characteristically play the key role in working with families in inpatient rehabilitation settings (Simpson et al., 2002), so it is relatively easier to investigate the impact of social work interventions, compared to clients with TBI who receive significant levels of intervention from all members of the multidisciplinary team. Second, the outcomes for families are of clinical importance, as families often play a critical role over the long term as the primary resource for the person with TBI (Barclay, 2013; Sander et al., 2003). Finally, many clients are still unconscious or in PTA when first admitted to the inpatient rehabilitation unit, and therefore, social workers often commence working with families from admission, whereas clients might not be able to participate until a later point during the episode of care.

In setting out to describe interventions delivered by social workers at the LBIRU, the example of previous studies that have characterized the social work role within other health settings were examined (e.g., renal dialysis, liver transplant, oncology, palliative care, cardiac care; Nilsson, Joubert, Holland, & Posenelli, 2013). In reviewing such studies, a predominant rationale was to demonstrate the organizational value of social work and to advocate for improved multidisciplinary practice (i.e., "what is done by hospital social workers and how other professions view hospital social workers'" Nilsson et al., 2013, p. 282). In contrast, this study aimed to "articulate social work practice more precisely" (Munro, 2004, p. 1085) as a means to then evaluate practice (Areán & Kraemer, 2013; Nilsson et al., 2013).

Approaches to describing interventions vary depending on whether one is developing a new intervention, adapting an intervention, or examining an existing intervention (Areán & Kraemer, 2013). In this case, the inpatient social work service to family members at the LBIRU had been continuously delivered by a number of social workers over a period of two decades, but still lacked a clear description of the key elements (Areán & Kraemer, 2013). Several approaches to describing the elements of social work activity in health settings have been reported, typically with a twin focus on the content of the intervention and the intensity or amount of time.

To document content, studies have developed purpose-designed classification systems drawing on previous literature (e.g., Judd & Sheffield, 2010) or accounts of interventions as outlined in social work textbooks (Bronstein, Kovacs, & Vega, 2007), adapted questionnaires from earlier studies (Kayser, Hansen, & Groves, 1995), or used existing departmental administrative systems that recorded daily social work activity (Davis, Baldry, Milosevic, & Walsh, 2004). To capture the time dimension, social work respondents have typically been asked to estimate the time allocated to their various roles or activities (e.g., Bronstein et al., 2007; Judd & Sheffield, 2010), with the exception of Davis et al. (2004), who retrospectively extracted actual time data from a departmental database. The advantage of such approaches is that they can be used to quickly capture data from large numbers of social workers practicing across a broad range of health settings. The disadvantages include the lack of any information about the reliability in both characterizing the content (i.e., how consistent was each social worker in classifying the same activities using the same categories) and in making the time estimates.

In seeking to describe existing psychosocial interventions in the field of brain injury, Hart (2009) recommended employing a coding approach. In this study, two code sets developed by the Australian National Allied Health Casemix Committee (Cleak, 2002) were used to delineate the content of the social work interventions. The National Allied Health Casemix Committee was an umbrella organization representing a range of allied health groups including social work, established and funded by the Australian federal government to respond to the growing spread of case mix funding approaches across the Australian health sector (Cleak, 2002). The National Allied Health Activity code set was developed to better characterize interventions by all allied health practices (including social work). Four broad categories were devised for all allied health activities, namely assessment and evaluation, counseling and education, case management and discharge planning, and other interventions. Each profession then developed specific intervention activities that fell within the four categories. The social work activity codes that were developed for the national framework and applied to categorize the LBIRU social work interventions are detailed in the Methods section of this article.

It is not sufficient, however, to simply describe the interventions. It is also important to identify the key problems and issues being addressed (Nilsson et al., 2013). Therefore, to complement the activity codes, a second code set, the indicators for intervention (IFIs), also developed by the National Allied Health Casemix Committee (1997), was employed. IFIs are defined as the trigger for intervention (Woodruff, Fitzgerland, & Itsiopoulos, 2000), providing information on the target for the intervention. Consistent with other classification systems (e.g., the International Classification of Diseases 10th Revision, Australian Modification [ICD–10–AM]), the IFIs were organized in a hierarchical system (Feltham, 2000). At the highest level (A level), there were two broad categories, namely person and environment. The next level, B level, outlined broad health and social issues, with the more specific codes most commonly used to describe social work services contained at the C and D levels (Cleak, 2002; see Results section for list of IFI codes). Therefore, the social work interventions delivered to families at the LBIRU were double coded (activities, IFIs).

However, in the original work done by the National Allied Health Casemix Committee, no system was devised for recording time against these two code sets (Cleak, 2002). Therefore, to maximize reliability in estimating service intensity in this study, time-based data for the social work services provided to families (both activity and IFI) were collected prospectively, using 15-min time units (e.g., Bronstein et al., 2007; Munro, 2004). Data were only collected on the clinical time in delivering services to families, including both direct and indirect service provision. Time-based data for nonclinical or nonpatient roles such as producing income, research, or administrative and departmental activities (e.g., Davis et al., 2004; Judd & Sheffield, 2010) were not collected.

In addition to being able to accurately characterize the social work intervention, the detailed description also provided the opportunity to examine the relative proportion of direct work (i.e., with the client) versus indirect work (i.e., with the client's environment; Butrym, 1968) provided by the LBIRU social workers. Studies in the United States have found that approximately 25% of social workers' time is spent on direct time (e.g., counseling, crisis intervention; Johnson, 1999; Judd & Sheffield, 2010), but in the Australian context, there are suggestions that the amount of direct work could be considerably higher (Davis et al., 2004; Nilsson et al., 2013). Understanding the ratio of direct to indirect services is an important element in crafting an evaluation approach, as it highlights where the social work interventions are focused.

The great majority of family intervention programs that have been published in the field of TBI have been developed by professions other than social work (e.g., nursing, psychology). Lechman, Sakadakis, and Tennier (2003) suggested that the distinctive characteristic of the social work role in the multidisciplinary team is the expertise to focus on both the social functioning and the environmental problems of the client. It was therefore telling that many of the published family interventions have had a predominantly person-centered focus, providing education only (e.g., Kreutzer, Marwitz, Sima, & Godwin, 2015; Powell, Fraser, Brockway, Temkin, & Bell, 2016; Sanguinetti & Catanzaro, 1987), education plus emotional support (Acorn, 1995; Brown et al., 1999), or therapeutic intervention only (Carnevale, 1996; Carnevale, Anselmi, Busichio, & Millis, 2002; Maitz & Sachs, 1995; Perlesz & O'Loughlan, 1998). In this study, the IFI codings with the basic person–environment division provided the opportunity to examine the balance of person-centered versus environment-centered interventions delivered by social work in comparison to these other published interventions.

This study employed an observational prospective longitudinal design to define the content and intensity of social work interventions for families during the inpatient phase of brain injury rehabilitation. By employing the national activity and IFI code sets, the study aimed to meet the conditions proposed by Nilsson et al. (2013) for defining meaningful outcome measures, namely "to accurately describe the nature of key problems/issues being addressed and the associated interventions" (p. 282). This study also provided the opportunity to investigate the balance of direct versus indirect time in the social work interventions.

Methods

Sample and service setting

The LBIRU is a regionally based, specialist brain injury rehabilitation unit that has a catchment population of approximately 1 million. It includes a 16-bed inpatient unit, a four-bed transitional living unit located 5 min from the hospital campus, a vocational rehabilitation service, a community rehabilitation team, and a four-bed residential respite service. The 20 beds (16 inpatient plus 4 transitional living) are covered by two full-time social workers, in accordance with the Standards for the Provision of Inpatient Rehabilitation of the Australasian Faculty of Rehabilitation Medicine (2011; one social worker per 10 inpatient beds for TBI). This study focused on the families of patients admitted to the 16 beds of the inpatient ward.

Australia has a universal health care system. All people who sustain a severe TBI, between the ages of 16 and 65, who are residents in the Sydney South West Local Health District are able to access the service. The LBIRU is part of the New South Wales Brain Injury Rehabilitation Program, a state-based network of 15 specialist brain injury rehabilitation services (Simpson, Sabaz, Daher, Gordon, & Strettles, 2014). The network is part of the state public health services and the majority provider of specialist brain injury rehabilitation within New South Wales. In the context of being a public health care service, the LBIRU has a needs-based approach to the provision of services, and discharge from the inpatient ward is determined on clinical grounds rather than insurance or other cost factors.

Approval for the study was granted by the Sydney South West Area Health Service Human Research Ethics Committee. A consecutive series of admissions to the inpatient unit from October 2005 and November 2006 were reviewed for their eligibility to participate in the study. Inclusion criteria included (a) family respondent was a first-degree relative of the person with TBI (e.g., parent, spouse, sibling, adult child); (b) relative sustained a de novo TBI between 18 and 65 years of age; (c) first admission to inpatient rehabilitation; (d) admission to inpatient rehabilitation unit within 6 months of injury; (e) one respondent per family; (f) admission longer than 2 weeks; and (f) family respondent does not have a current psychiatric illness.

A total of 27 families participated in the study. Another 21 families were admitted to the inpatient unit during the recruitment period but did not meet the inclusion criteria (multiple head injuries $n = 4$, short admission less than 2 weeks $n = 10$, no next of kin $n = 2$, limited English fluency $n = 4$, and psychiatric illness $n = 1$). Finally, 6 families who met the inclusion criteria declined to participate. Demographic and injury data for the participating family members and their relative with TBI are presented in Table 1. Family members were generally female. The relationships for the majority of participants to

Table 1. Demographic and injury details.

Variable	Data
Family member	
Sex (n, %)	
Male	10, 37
Female	17, 63
Relationship to person with TBI (n, %)	
Parent	13, 49
Spouse	9, 33
Adult child	2, 7
Adult sibling	3, 11
Age (years) at interview (M, SD)	49, 9
Education (years) (M, SD)	12, 5
Living with person with TBI at injury (yes) (n, %)	20, 74
Person with TBI	
Sex (n, %)	
Male	19, 70
Female	8, 30
Cause of injury (n, %)	
Road	17, 63
Other (fall, assault)	10, 37
Severity of injury	
GCS (lowest in first 24hr) (M, SD)	6, 4
PTA (days) (med, IQR)	55, 45
Age at injury (years) (M, SD)	36, 15
Time from injury to admission (days) (M, SD)	53, 24
Length of stay (weeks) (M, SD)	12, 20

Note: n=27. TBI=traumatic brain injury; GCS=Glasgow Coma Scale; PTA=posttraumatic amnesia; IQR=interquartile range.

the person with TBI were as a parent or spouse. Three quarters of the family members had been living with the person with TBI at the time of the injury. Some background information was also collected about the person with TBI to provide context to the challenges facing the family members. The majority were relatively young men who had sustained extremely severe injuries, predominantly as the result of road accidents, the typical injury profile for people sustaining TBIs of this severity. Not surprisingly, the corresponding average duration of stay in the inpatient rehabilitation unit was quite lengthy (i.e., 12 weeks).

Measures

Data collection involved the use of a purpose-designed data protocol and the two coding sets. The data protocol was devised to collect demographic, injury, and psychosocial information about the participating family member and his or her relatives with TBI.

Coding sets

Two coding systems were employed to address the study aim. The Allied Health Activity Codes are part of the Australian Allied Health Classification

System codes (National Allied Health Casemix Committee, 1997), which form a chapter covering 11 allied health disciplines within the ICD–10–AM. As highlighted earlier, the four generic allied health activities specified in this coding system were (a) assessment and evaluation, (b) counseling and education, (c) case management and discharge planning, and (d) other interventions. Social work generated 13 activity codes within these four overarching categories. The 11 codes from the list employed for the current project were (a) psychosocial assessment; (b) counseling, crisis intervention, and education; (c) case management and discharge planning, service coordination, liaison, referring, and resourcing; and (d) advocacy and other interventions. In this study, other interventions were elaborated, introducing guardianship (appointing substitute or proxy decision makers) and conflict resolution, as well as an "other" category to catch any other activities not already recorded. Guardianship and conflict resolution were introduced based on clinical experience, resulting in a total of 13 activity codes.

Bereavement counseling and critical incident stress debriefing (the other available codes) were not included, because neither type of intervention was generally employed in the inpatient rehabilitation setting. Critical incident stress debriefing was more likely to occur in acute medical settings, and bereavement counseling is more commonly provided during the long-term community phase, as most families have a recovery-oriented focus during the inpatient episode of care.

The IFI coding system provided data on the clinical issues that were the target of the social work intervention. The IFI codes were interdisciplinary (i.e., issues that could potentially be addressed by more than one discipline). Because the codes were part of the ICS–10–AM, they covered 11 allied health disciplines, and a broad range of codes were developed (Cleak, 2002). Therefore, the IFI code set was reviewed by the authors and a subset was selected that was applicable to social work, principally from among the D level codes (which provide the most detailed descriptor of the presenting clinical issue), except for some codes that were defined at the C level with no D codes.

Procedures

Data collection

All family members of relatives admitted to the LBIRU inpatient service who met the inclusion criteria during the study period were invited to take part. Participants were volunteers and provided informed consent. Information was then collected for the participant data protocol.

Occasions of service were collected in 15-min units of time. Therefore a 1-hr family meeting would be coded as four occasions of service. A data template was devised for the authors to record the coding of the occasions of service using both the activity and IFI classification systems. Each activity coding unit was also classified as direct or 'indirect. Direct services included face-to-face or phone interactions with one or more family members. Indirect services included phoning a third party on behalf of the family, such as a service provider.

During the data collection phase, the research team held regular meetings to monitor the coding and make consensus decisions around occasions of service that were difficult to code. In addition to the coding sets, data were collected on the number of family members who attended formal or informal meetings with the social worker, the actual number of formal and informal meetings held, and the number of meetings conducted with an interpreter (all accredited New South Wales Health interpreters).

Social work intervention

The social work interventions were provided by two graduate social workers with 4 and 9 years of experience. The approach to social work interventions in the LBIRU inpatient unit was learned in vivo, through supervision from the LBIRU social work team leader and mentoring from other social workers who had previously worked in the inpatient setting. The social work interventions were needs based, and did not involve a manualized program.

The social workers organized and chaired the formal meetings between family members, their relatives, and the multidisciplinary team, which were held at set times during the inpatient episode of care and were a key channel for the communication of information between the team and the family (e.g., first week with doctor and social worker for orientation; a second meeting with the larger multidisciplinary team for feedback on the results of assessments; and a further meeting with the larger multidisciplinary team with a focus on discharge planning later during the episode of care). For patients with longer stays, additional progress meetings with the larger multidisciplinary team might also be held.

Social workers also held a number of informal meetings with family members to address the broader range of issues encountered by the families that fell within the scope of the social work role. These meetings were the primary means by which information provision and counseling were provided. The social work approach was systemic in nature, seeking to engage as many family members as possible and including them in the process of supporting their relatives during the inpatient rehabilitation phase. The social work interventions were delivered at the center, with home visits or community agency visits rare. Case management, most commonly discharge planning, was conducted through direct contact (face-to-face meetings, phone contacts) with the family members, as well as through accessing community-based service providers (both government and nongovernment), who were to provide support to the family and their relatives postdischarge.

Data analysis

Data were entered into SPSS 22. A kappa statistic was calculated to assess the reliability of the activities coding. Following Landis and Koch (1977), a kappa statistic of .21 to .40 was interpreted as representing fair agreement, .41 to .60 moderate agreement, and .61 to .80 substantial agreement. Descriptive statistics were generated for the activity and IFI codes. For ease of interpretation the occasions of service were aggregated into hours.

Results

Overall summary of family intervention

A total of 655 hr of service data were analyzed for the 27 participating families. On average, families received 24 hr of service (see Table 2), with a total of 79 family members seen at least once. For every hour that family members spent in a formal multidisciplinary team meeting, they received another 4 hr of intervention in informal meetings with the social worker.

Interrater reliability analysis

A reliability analysis was conducted to check the accuracy of the coding for the social work interventions (activities). The kappa statistic for paired ratings on the first 34 occasions of service was calculated ($\kappa = .71$, $p < .001$). The result indicated that there was a substantial level of agreement in the approach to coding the interventions between the two social workers.

Activities code set

Examining the proportions of the different classes of activity codes, the three most common services provided by social workers were education and information, case management, and counseling, as shown in Table 3. Overall, the person-centered interventions (assessment, counseling, crisis management, education and information, conflict resolution) accounted for about 50% of all occasions of service. The balance of the time was focused on

Table 2. Overview of services provided to families.

Variable	Data		
	M	SD	Range
Number of family members seen per family[a]	3	1	1–6
Formal meetings	3	2	0–6
Informal meetings	12	8	2–32
Hours of family support	24	19	6–88
Interpreter use ($n = 4$) (hr)	12	9	5–25

Note: $n = 27$.
[a]Total of 79 family members seen.

Table 3. Social work activities (Hr).

Activity	Direct	Indirect	% total hours
Assessment	40	1	6%
Counseling	113	—	17%
Crisis management	21	2	4%
Education/information	149	3	23%
Case management/discharge planning	103	24	19%
Service coordination	5	3	1%
Liaison	7	40	7%
Referral	9	8	3%
Resourcing	15	22	6%
Advocacy	13	22	5%
Guardianship	12	15	4%
Conflict resolution	25	—	4%
Other	2	1	1%
Total hours	514	141	100%

Note: n = 27.

environment-centered interventions, with discharge planning the most frequent component of the case management activity code documented.

Analyzing the average hours of service provision per family, the amount of indirect service required for the person-centered interventions was negligible (direct hours $= 13.0 \pm 10.0$; indirect hours $= 0.5 \pm 0.4$). In contrast, work on environment-centered interventions required a different approach. Almost half of the work in this domain comprised indirect hours (direct hours $= 6.0 \pm 6.0$; indirect hours $= 5.0 \pm 6.0$), involving the liaison or advocacy with service providers and service systems on behalf of the family.

Indicators for intervention code set

The data from the IFI codes provided information on the range of clinical issues that triggered social work intervention (see Table 4). The most common person-centered IFI codes were systemic interpersonal issues (i.e., supporting family members in adapting to the changed relationship with their relatives who had sustained the TBI) and adjustment to health (i.e., providing education to families about brain injury). IFIs for the environment spanned transport, legal, accommodation, finances, citizenship, insurance, and guardianship. This reflected the complexity and wide-ranging nature of family issues after TBI. Families typically had identified multiple issues that needed to be addressed concurrently.

Discussion

This study has provided a detailed description of the program of social work interventions provided within an inpatient brain injury rehabilitation unit for the first time. In doing so, it has helped to unpack the black box of social work

Table 4. Indicator for intervention codes.

Indicator for intervention	Examples	Total hours	
		n	%
Person			
Cognition	Education about posttraumatic amnesia	31	5
Interpersonal (parent, partner, systemic, abuse)	Assessment of family system, managing family system as a whole	147	23
Social conduct	Social work providing support to family who are the target of verbal abuse, etc.	21	3
Adjustment to health	Education about brain injury	151	23
Adjustment to hospital	Education about hospital/LBIRU procedures	53	8
Bereavement	Support if some related family member or friend died in the accident	3	1
Affect (anxiety and mood)	Heightened levels of anxiety related to rehabilitation progress, discharge	16	2
Environment			
Productivity (work, study, home duties)		16	2
Environment		215	33
Transport	Parking vouchers, disability vouchers, taxi vouchers, transport for appointments		
Legal	Legal advice to address compensation, access lawyers, accessing legal aide regarding criminal matters, court reports		
Accommodation	Apply for housing; identify group homes; identifying other accommodation options		
Finance/resources	Bank accounts, superannuation, apply for financial assistance in relation to debts, apply for income support		
Citizenship	Immigration, bring family to visit, injured illegal immigrants, apply to extend visas		
Insurance	Accessing compensation, compensation rights		
Guardianship	Substitute decision making, power of attorney, applications for guardian or financial orders		
Total		653	100

Note: $n = 27$. LBIRU = Liverpool Brain Injury Rehabilitation Unit.

intervention (Munro, 2004) within this setting, thereby addressing in part the broader challenge faced by brain injury units in unpacking the black box of neurorehabilitation programs more generally (Hart, 2009; Whyte & Hart, 2003). Three major areas of social work activity were identified, namely education and information, counseling, and case management (predominantly discharge planning). The reliability check suggested that the coding of the social work interventions was conducted with a high degree of reliability.

The program is novel in the field of TBI in three regards. First, to the best of our knowledge, this is the first description of a program targeting families in the inpatient rehabilitation setting. Within the context of the published programs focusing on the postacute phase, the social work services detailed in this study could be characterized as an early intervention program. The second novel aspect is the intensity of the program. The average of 24 hr of intervention per family is at the upper limit for the published programs (i.e., 15–20 hr; Brown et al., 1999; Sinnakaruppan, Downey, & Morrison,

2005). It is also triple the time reported by Davis et al. (2004) within the Australian context for hospital-based social work services more generally. This difference could be explained in part by the setting; patients have substantial lengths of stay in the inpatient rehabilitation context compared to patients in general hospital wards.

Third, the program is also novel in the integration of person-centered and environment-centered interventions, as documented both in the activities and the IFI codes. The environment-centered needs were principally addressed through the case management intervention (specifically discharge planning). Although the need for environmental supports for families has been identified in the literature, including legal and financial problems (Albert, Im, Brenner, Smith, & Waxman, 2002; Hall et al., 1994), accommodation (Brzuzy & Speziale, 1997), and citizenship and immigration (e.g., Simpson, Mohr, & Redman, 2000), the greatest extent to which the published family interventions have addressed such issues (if at all) has been to include information about available community services (e.g., Kreutzer et al., 2015). The one exception to this is the only previously published social work program (Albert et al., 2002) that involved following up with families to link them into services postdischarge from the inpatient brain injury rehabilitation service. This important contribution of social work to discharge planning reflects the findings from a number of other studies both within TBI (e.g., Levesque, 1988) and the health sector more generally (Davis et al., 2004; Judd & Sheffield, 2010).

More broadly, this focus on environment reflects an important dimension of the World Health Organization [WHO] International Classification of Functioning, Disability and Health (ICF; WHO, 2001) framework. The ICF recognizes that characteristics of the person and the environment are both contextual factors that influence the well-being and outcomes of individuals with health conditions (Barrow, 2006), including the individual with TBI (Bernabeu et al., 2009). These same concepts can also be applied to the well-being and outcomes for families supporting relatives with TBI.

The other two main areas of social work activity were information and education and counseling. Starting with the former, a number of programs providing information for families after TBI have been documented (Acorn, 1995; Brown et al., 1999; Kreutzer et al., 2015; Powell et al., 2016; Sanguinetti & Catanzaro, 1987), but to the best of our knowledge, this study provides the first description of such intervention to address the information and education needs of families within an inpatient setting. No systematic reviews have been conducted looking at best practice for information provision to families in TBI. However, such a review has demonstrated the efficacy of information provision for families caring for a relative with stroke (Forster et al., 2004). Of particular interest, the strongest evidence in terms of the mode of delivery was found for approaches that maximized the degree of interaction between family members and staff in processing the information. The needs-based and individualized approach that the LBIRU social workers employ in providing information and education to families at the LBIRU is consistent with such an approach. Further indirect support can be found for the efficacy of another element of the LBIRU social work role in the area of information and education, namely the organization and chairing of the family conferences. A recent systematic review has found moderate evidence for the efficacy of such family meetings in reducing psychological distress and increasing knowledge about broader health conditions among family members (Reed & Harding, 2015).

The other area of social work activity was counseling. As outlined earlier, adjustment to the hospital setting and to the health condition, as well as anxiety and depression, were significant IFIs for social work. The focus on adjustment in the person-oriented domain suggested that counseling complemented information and education as an intervention to facilitate adjustment, in line with the predominantly recovery-oriented focus of families toward their relatives during the inpatient phase (Baker et al., 2002; Simpson et al., 2002). Although a decision was made to not include bereavement in the activity code set, the one instance in which bereavement counseling was provided was captured by the IFI codes. This related to bereavement counseling provided to one family mourning the loss of a close family friend who died in the same accident that left their own relative with a severe TBI. Given the number of road accidents that involve multiple occupants within vehicles with the potential for fatalities, the data suggest that there might be an occasional need for bereavement-related interventions during the inpatient rehabilitation phase.

The IFIs in the person-centered domain highlighted the focus on relationships. The systemic nature of the program was reflected in the number of family members who received social work intervention. This systemic focus is important, because previous research has documented a range of needs among multiple family members and not just a "primary caregiver" (e.g., Charles, Butera-Prinzi, & Perlesz, 2007; Degeneffe & Olney, 2008; Perlesz et al., 2000).

The study also examined whether patient attributable work included non-direct clinical activities or was restricted to direct face-to-face clinical time (Cleak, 2002). Results showed that the proportion of direct versus indirect service provision varied depending on the type of intervention. The person-oriented interventions such as counseling and information and education required very little indirect time. By contrast, the environment-oriented interventions required as much indirect time as direct hours. This has important implications in terms of service documentation. If health services or other organizations only collect service activity data or only bill for face-to-face hours, the true cost of addressing the environmental needs of families and their relatives ends up being hidden, with the possible restrictions of the extent to which such services can be provided.

This study has laid the groundwork for evaluation of the program in being able to select outcome measures that will assess the areas targeted by the social work interventions. Although in the National Allied Health code set, the IFIs were flagged as providing the platform for defining outcomes, this was never acted on (Cleak, 2002). However, social work can draw on existing outcome measures within the field of TBI to evaluate the outcomes from the social work interventions.

Previous published family intervention studies have employed a range of instruments including the Profile of Mood States (POMS; McNair, Lorr, & Droppleman, 1981), the General Health Questionnaire–28 (Goldberg & Williams, 1988), and the Family Assessment Device (Epstein, Bishop, & Levin, 1978), among others, to assess psychological distress and family functioning (e.g., Brown et al., 1999; Perlesz & O'Loughlan, 1998; Sinnakaruppan et al., 2005), and these types of measures could be employed to evaluate outcomes from social work. Evaluating the efficacy of information provision is challeng-ing because few scales exist within the field of TBI to measure this area, however the POMS does have a subscale (Confusion) that taps into this domain. Fewer measures are currently available to assess the impact of changes to the environment. However, the Medical Outcomes Scale of Social Support (Sherbourne & Stewart, 1991) has been frequently used to evaluate the degree of social support available to families and the Service Obstacles Scale (Kreutzer, 2000) has been used in family intervention studies (i.e., Kreutzer et al., 2015; Kreutzer et al., 2009) and could help to quantify barriers requiring social work advocacy. In addition, new measures have been developed that are aligned with the ICF Environment domain (e.g., the Craig Hospital Inventory of Environmental Factors; Whiteneck et al., 2004) that might help to capture data about important areas of social work activity.

In introducing any evaluation measures, the issue of timing of administra-tion is important. Immediate impact could be assessed by administration of measures at admission and discharge to the inpatient ward. However, in seeking to evaluate outcomes, the importance of systematically monitoring outcomes over the longer term has also been flagged (Cleak, 2002; Munro, 2004). The suggestion is that people receiving social work interventions in the inpatient setting might experience a delayed benefit rather than an immediate impact that is measurable at the point the social work intervention ceases, and highlights the need for longer term follow-up.

The limitations of the study need to be acknowledged. First, it reports on data from a single center and might not generalize to the profile of social work interventions delivered in other inpatient brain injury rehabilitation centers, particularly ones in other countries. Next, although the social workers were the key workers with the family members, all members of the multidisci-plinary team had some interaction with families, particularly in the structured family meetings. Furthermore, the multidisciplinary staff involved in the dis-charge planning process also played critical roles in some of the environ-ment-related interventions. It was not possible to document the informal interactions of all team members with the families, and if this additional data had been collected, it might have influenced the balance of the results.

Overall, the social work interventions at the LBIRU could be characterized as an intensive family psychosocial support program. By specifying the program in some detail, these findings lay the foundation for several lines of inquiry. Future research could examine whether an "early intervention" program delivered within the inpatient setting reduces the level of distress experienced by families over the longer term. Next, the coding set for activities was still fairly general, and provided little indication about the content needed for education and information or the types of counseling that were provided (e.g., supportive counseling, adjustment counseling, cognitive-behavior therapy, family counseling); further work could be done to elicit this information. Developing new measures to capture the efficacy of interventions that focus on mobilizing environment-related supports in contributing to the overall well-being of families is also important. For example, the utility of the social work developed Assessment of Living and Resources scale (ALSAR; Williams et al., 1991) in partialing out the relative contribution of person-centered versus environment-centered interventions in promoting independence for people with TBI has been demonstrated (Simpson et al., 2004). The concepts underlying the design of this measure could serve as a model for developing new measures to assess the outcomes of interventions with family members.

In conclusion, this study provided a detailed breakdown of the social work interventions that have been conducted with families within the inpatient rehabilitation setting. It lays the groundwork for future evaluation that can accurately assess the outcomes from the treatments provided. The hope is that this will be a win–win, benefiting both the family caregivers of people with TBI and the social work profession.

References

Access Economics. (2008). *The economic cost of spinal cord injury and traumatic brain injury in Australia*. Melbourne, Australia: Victorian Neurotrauma Institute.

Acorn, S. (1995). Assisting families of head-injured survivors through a family support program. *Journal of Advanced Nursing, 21,* 872–877. doi:10.1046/j.1365-2648.1995.21050872.x

Albert, S. M., Im, A., Brenner, L., Smith, M., & Waxman, R. (2002). Effect of a social work liaison program on family caregivers to people with brain injury. *Journal of Head Trauma Rehabilitation, 17,* 175–189. doi:10.1097/00001199-200204000-00007

Anderson, M. I., Simpson, G. K., & Morey, P. J. (2013). The impact of neurobehavioural impairment on family functioning and the psychological wellbeing of male versus female caregivers of relatives with severe traumatic brain injury: Multi-group analysis. *Journal of Head Trauma Rehabilitation, 28,* 453–463. doi:10.1097/HTR.0b013e31825d6087

Anderson, M. I., Simpson, G. K., Morey, P. J., Mok, M., Gosling, T. J., & Gillett, L. E. (2009). Differential pathways of psychological distress in spouses versus parents of people with severe traumatic brain injury (TBI): Multigroup analysis. *Brain Injury, 23,* 931–943. doi:10.3109/02699050903302336

Areán, P. A., & Kraemer, H. C. (2013). *High quality psychotherapy research: From conception to piloting to national trials*. Oxford, UK: Oxford University Press.

Australasian Faculty of Rehabilitation Medicine. (2011). *Standards for the provision of inpatient adult rehabilitation medical services in public and private hospitals*. Sydney, Australia: Author.

Baker, K. A., Tandy, C. C., & Dixon, D. R. (2002). Traumatic brain injury: A social work primer. *Journal of Social Work in Disability and Rehabilitation, 1,* 25–44. doi:10.1300/J198v01n04_03

Barclay, D. A. (2013). Family functioning, psychosocial stress, and goal attainment in brain injury rehabilitation. *Journal of Social Work in Disability & Rehabilitation, 12,* 159–175. doi:10.1080/1536710X.2013.810093

Barrow, F. H. (2006). The international classification of functioning, disability, and health (ICF): A new tool for social workers. *Journal of Social Work in Disability and Rehabilitation, 5,* 65–73.

Bernabeu, M., Laxe, S., Lopez, R., Stucki, G., Ward, A., Barnes, M., … Cieza, A. (2009). Developing core sets for persons with traumatic brain injury based on the international classification of functioning, disability and health. *Neurorehabilitation and Neural Repair, 23,* 464–467. doi:10.1177/1545968308328725

Bronstein, L., Kovacs, P., & Vega, A. (2007). Goodness of fit: Social work education and practice in health care. *Social Work in Health Care, 45*(2), 59–76. doi:10.1300/J010v45n02_04

Brown, A., Pain, K., Berwald, C., Hirschi, P., Delehanty, R., & Miller, H. (1999). Distance education and caregiver support groups: Comparison of traditional and telephone groups. *Journal of Head Trauma Rehabilitation, 14,* 257–268. doi:10.1097/00001199-199906000-00006

Brzuzy, S., & Speziale, B. A. (1997). Persons with traumatic brain injuries and their families: Living arrangements and well-being post injury. *Social Work in Health Care, 26*(1), 77–88. doi:10.1300/J010v26n01_05

Butrym, Z. (1968). *Medical social work in action*. London, UK: Bell and Sons.

Carlton, T. O., & Stephenson, M. D. G. (1990). Social work and the management of severe head injury. *Social Science & Medicine, 31*(1), 5–11. doi:10.1016/0277-9536(90)90003-B

Carnevale, G. J. (1996). Natural-setting behavior management for individuals with traumatic brain injury: Results of a three-year caregiver training program. *The Journal of Head Trauma Rehabilitation, 11*(1), 27–38. doi:10.1097/00001199-199602000-00005

Carnevale, G. J., Anselmi, V., Busichio, K., & Millis, S. R. (2002). Changes in ratings of caregiver burden following a community-based behavior management program for persons with traumatic brain injury. *The Journal of Head Trauma Rehabilitation, 17*(2), 83–95. doi:10.1097/00001199-200204000-00002

Chambless, D. L., & Hollon, S. D. (1998). Defining empirically supported therapies. *Journal of Consulting and Clinical Psychology, 66*(1), 7. doi:10.1037/0022-006X.66.1.7

Charles, N., Butera-Prinzi, F., & Perlesz, A. (2007). Families living with acquired brain injury: A multiple family group experience. *NeuroRehabilitation, 22*(1), 61–76.

Cleak, H. (2002). A model of social work classification in health care. *Australian Social Work, 55*(1), 38–49. doi:10.1080/03124070208411670

Daisley, A., Tams, R., & Kischka, U. (2009). *Head injury*. Oxford, UK: Oxford University Press.

Davis, C., Baldry, E., Milosevic, B., & Walsh, A. (2004). Defining the role of the hospital social worker in Australia. *International Social Work, 47*, 346–358. doi:10.1177/0020872804043958

Degeneffe, C. E. (2001). Family caregiving and traumatic brain injury. *Health and Social Work, 26*, 257–268. doi:10.1093/hsw/26.4.257

Degeneffe, C. E., & Olney, M. F. (2008). Future concerns of adult siblings of persons with traumatic brain injury. *Rehabilitation Counselling Bulletin, 51*, 240–250. doi:10.1177/0034355207311319

Epstein, N. B., Bishop, D. S., & Levin, S. (1978). The McMaster model of family functioning. *Journal of Marriage and Family Counselling, 4*, 19–31. doi:10.1111/j.1752-0606.1978.tb00537.x

Feltham, C. (2000). Counselling supervision: Baselines, problems and possibilities. In B. Lawton, & C. Feltham (Eds.), *Taking supervision forward: Enquiries and trends in counselling and psychotherapy*, (pp. 5–24). London, UK: Sage.

Forster, A., Smith, J., Young, J., Knapp, P., House, A., & Wright, J. (2004). Information provision for stroke patients and their caregivers (Cochrane review). *The Cochrane Library, 1*, 1–74.

Frost, R. B., Farrer, T. J., Primosch, M., & Hedges, D. W. (2013). Prevalence of traumatic brain injury in the general adult population: A meta-analysis. *Neuroepidemiology, 40*, 154–159. doi:10.1159/000343275

Goldberg, D., & Williams, P. (1988). *A user's guide to the general health questionnaire*. Windsor, UK: NFER-Nelson.

Hall, K. M., Karzmark, P., Stevens, M., Englander, J., O'Hare, P., & Wright, J. (1994). Family stressors in traumatic brain injury: A two-year follow-up. *Archives of Physical Medicine and Rehabilitation, 75*, 876–884. doi:10.1016/0003-9993(94)90112-0

Hart, T. (2009). Treatment definition in complex rehabilitation interventions. *Neuropsychological Rehabilitation, 19*, 824–840. doi:10.1080/09602010902995945

Johnson, Y. M. (1999). Indirect work: Social work's uncelebrated strength. *Social Work, 44*, 323–334. doi:10.1093/sw/44.4.323

Judd, R. G., & Sheffield, S. (2010). Hospital social work: Contemporary roles and professional activities. *Social Work in Health Care, 49*, 856–871. doi:10.1080/00981389.2010.499825

Kayser, K., Hansen, P., & Groves, A. (1995). Evaluating social work practice in a medical setting: How do we meet the challenges of a rapidly changing system? *Research on Social Work Practice, 5*, 485–500. doi:10.1177/104973159500500407

Khan, F., Baguley, I. J., & Cameron, I. D. (2003). 4: Rehabilitation after traumatic brain injury. *Medical Journal of Australia, 178*, 290–297.

Kreutzer, J. S. (2000). *The Service Obstacles Scale*. The Center for Outcome Measurement in Brain Injury. Retrieved from http://www.tbims.org/combi/sos

Kreutzer, J. S., Marwitz, J. H., Sima, A. P., & Godwin, E. E. (2015). Efficacy of the brain injury family intervention: Impact on family members. *Journal of Head Trauma Rehabilitation, 30*, 249–260. doi:10.1097/HTR.0000000000000144

Kreutzer, J. S., Rapport, L. J., Marwitz, J. H., Harrison-Felix, C., Hart, T., Glenn, M., & Hammond, F. (2009). Caregivers' well-being after traumatic brain injury: A multicenter prospective investigation. *Archives of Physical Medicine and Rehabilitation, 90*, 939–946. doi:10.1016/j.apmr.2009.01.010

Landis, J. R., & Koch, G. G. (1977). The measurement of observer agreement for categorical data. *Biometrics, 33*, 159–174. doi:10.2307/2529310

Langlois, J. A., Rutland-Brown, W., & Wald, M. M. (2006). The epidemiology and impact of traumatic brain injury: A brief overview. *Journal of Head Trauma Rehabilitation, 21*, 375–378. doi:10.1097/00001199-200609000-00001

Lechman, C., Sakadakis, V., & Tennier, L. (2003). PIE: A tool for defining the role of social work in a multi-disciplinary hospital. *Intervention: Travailleurs Sociaux, Multidisciplinarite et Interdiciplinarite, 18*(July), 15–20.

Levesque, J. D. (1988). Assessing the foreseeable risks in discharge planning: The challenge of discharging the brain-injured patient. *Social Work in Health Care, 13*, 49–63. doi:10.1300/J010v13n04_05

Lezak, M. D. (1988). Brain damage is a family affair. *Journal of Clinical and Experimental Neuropsychology, 10*, 111–123. doi:10.1080/01688638808405098

Livingston, M. G., Brooks, D. N., & Bond, M. R. (1985). Patient outcome in the year following severe head injury and relatives' psychiatric and social functioning. *Journal of Neurology, Neurosurgery, & Psychiatry, 48*, 876–881. doi:10.1136/jnnp.48.9.876

Maitz, E. A., & Sachs, P. R. (1995). Treating families of individuals with traumatic brain injury from a family systems perspective. *Journal of Head Trauma Rehabilitation, 10*, 1–11. doi:10.1097/00001199-199504000-00003

Marsh, N. V., Kersel, D. A., Havill, J. H., & Sleigh, J. W. (1998). Caregiver burden at 6 months following severe traumatic brain injury. *Brain Injury, 12*, 225–238. doi:10.1080/026990598122700

McNair, D. M., Lorr, M., & Droppleman, L. F. (1981). *Profile of Mood States*. San Diego, CA: Educational and Industrial Testing Service.

Munro, E. (2004). The impact of audit on social work practice. *British Journal of Social Work, 34*, 1075–1095. doi:10.1093/bjsw/bch130

National Allied Health Casemix Committee. (1997). *Australian Allied Health Classification System, Version 1*. Melbourne, Australia: Author.

Nilsson, D., Joubert, L., Holland, L., & Posenelli, S. (2013). The why of practice: Utilizing PIE to analyze social work practice in Australian hospitals. *Social Work in Health Care, 52*, 280–295. doi:10.1080/00981389.2012.737901

Peeters, W., van den Brande, R., Polinder, S., Brazinova, A., Steyerberg, E. W., Lingsma, H. F., & Maas, A. I. (2015). Epidemiology of traumatic brain injury in Europe. *Acta Neurochirurgica, 157*, 1683–1696. doi:10.1007/s00701-015-2512-7

Perlesz, A., Kinsella, G., & Crowe, S. (2000). Psychological distress and family satisfaction following traumatic brain injury: Injured individuals and their primary, secondary and tertiary carers. *Journal of Head Trauma Rehabilitation, 15*, 909–929. doi:10.1097/00001199-200006000-00005

Perlesz, A., & O'Loughlan, M. (1998). Changes in stress and burden in families seeking therapy following traumatic brain injury: A follow-up study. *International Journal of Rehabilitation Research, 21,* 339–354. doi:10.1097/00004356-199812000-00001

Powell, J. M., Fraser, R., Brockway, J. A., Temkin, N., & Bell, K. R. (2016). A telehealth approach to caregiver self-management following traumatic brain injury: A randomized controlled trial. *Journal of Head Trauma Rehabilitation, 31,* 180–190. doi:10.1097/HTR.0000000000000167

Reed, M., & Harding, K. E. (2015). Do family meetings improve measurable outcomes for patients, carers, or health systems? A systematic review. *Australian Social Work, 68,* 244–258. doi:10.1080/0312407X.2014.913070

Rosen, A., Proctor, E. K., & Staudt, M. M. (1999). Social work research and the quest for effective practice. *Social Work Research, 23*(1), 4–14. doi:10.1093/swr/23.1.4

Royse, D. (2008). *Research methods in social work,* (5th ed.). Belmont, CA: Thomson Higher Education.

Russell, W. R., & Smith, A. (1961). Post-traumatic amnesia in closed head injury. *Archives of Neurology, 5,* 4–17. doi:10.1001/archneur.1961.00450130006002

Sander, A. M., Maestas, K. L., Clark, A. N., & Havins, W. N. (2013). Predictors of emotional distress in family caregivers of persons with traumatic brain injury: A systematic review. *Brain Impairment, 14,* 113–129. doi:10.1017/BrImp.2013.12

Sander, A. M., Sherer, M., Malec, J. F., High, W. M., Jr., Thompson, R. N., Moessner, A. M., & Josey, J. (2003). Preinjury emotional and family functioning in caregivers of persons with traumatic brain injury. *Archives of Physical Medicine and Rehabilitation, 84,* 197–203. doi:10.1053/apmr.2003.50105

Sanguinetti, M., & Catanzaro, M. (1987). A comparison of discharge teaching on the consequences of brain injury. *Journal of Neuroscience Nursing, 19,* 271–275. doi:10.1097/01376517-198710000-00010

Sherbourne, C. D., & Stewart, A. L. (1991). The MOS social support survey. *Social Science and Medicine, 32,* 705–714. doi:10.1016/0277-9536(91)90150-B

Simpson, G. K., Mohr, R., & Redman, A. (2000). Cultural variations in the understanding of traumatic brain injury and brain injury rehabilitation. *Brain Injury, 14,* 125–140. doi:10.1080/026990500120790

Simpson, G. K., Sabaz, M., Daher, M., Gordon, R., & Strettles, B. (2014). Service utilisation and service access among community-dwelling clients with challenging behaviours after severe traumatic brain injury: A multicentre study. *Brain Impairment, 15,* 28–42. doi:10.1017/BrImp.2014.7

Simpson, G. K., Secheny, T., Lane-Brown, A., Strettles, B., Ferry, K., & Phillips, J. (2004). Post-acute rehabilitation for people with traumatic brain injury: A model description and evaluation of the Liverpool hospital transitional living program. *Brain Impairment, 5,* 67–80. doi:10.1375/brim.5.1.67.35401

Simpson, G. K., Simons, M., & McFadyen, M. (2002). The challenges of a hidden disability: Social work practice in the field of traumatic brain injury. *Australian Social Work, 55,* 24–37. doi:10.1080/03124070208411669

Sinnakaruppan, I., Downey, B., & Morrison, S. (2005). Head injury and family carers: A pilot study to investigate an innovative community-based education programme for family carers and patients. *Brain Injury, 19,* 283–308. doi:10.1080/02699050400003924

Tate, R. L., McDonald, S., & Lulham, J. M. (1998). Incidence of hospital-treated traumatic brain injury in an Australian community. *Australian and New Zealand Journal of Public Health, 22,* 419–423. doi:10.1111/j.1467-842X.1998.tb01406.x

Teasdale, G. M. (1995). Head injury. *Journal of Neurology, Neurosurgery, & Psychiatry, 58,* 526–539. doi:10.1136/jnnp.58.5.526

Tverdov, A. H., McClure, K. S., Brownsberger, M. G., & Armstrong, S. L. (2016). Family needs at a post-acute rehabilitation setting and suggestions for supports. *Brain Injury*, *30*, 324–333. doi:10.3109/02699052.2015.1113566

Warden, D. (2006). Military TBI during the Iraq and Afghanistan wars. *Journal of Head Trauma Rehabilitation*, *21*, 398–402. doi:10.1097/00001199-200609000-00004

Whiteneck, G., Meade, M. A., Dijkers, M., Tate, D. G., Bushnik, T., & Forchheimer, M. B. (2004). Environmental factors and their role in participation and life satisfaction after spinal cord injury. *Archives of Physical Medicine and Rehabilitation*, *85*, 1793–1803. doi:10.1016/j.apmr.2004.04.024

Whyte, J., & Hart, T. (2003). It's more than a black box; It's a Russian doll: Defining rehabilitation treatments. *American Journal of Physical Medicine & Rehabilitation*, *82*, 639–652. doi:10.1097/01.PHM.0000078200.61840.2D

Williams, J. H., Drinka, T. J. K., Greenberg, J. R., Farrell-Holtan, J., Euhardy, R., & Schram, M. (1991). Development and testing of the assessment of living skills and resources (ALSAR) in elderly community-dwelling veterans. *The Gerontologist*, *31*, 84–91. doi:10.1093/geront/31.1.84

Winstanley, J., Simpson, G. K., Tate, R. L., & Miles, B. (2006). Early indicators and causal factors of psychological distress in relatives during rehabilitation following severe TBI: Findings from the brain injury outcomes study. *Journal of Head Trauma Rehabilitation*, *21*, 453–466. doi:10.1097/00001199-200611000-00001

Woodruff, I., Fitzgerland, K., & Itsiopoulos, C. (2000) *Report on the development of allied health indicators for intervention (IFI) and performance indicators (PI) and revision of allied health-sensitive ICD–10–AM codes for inclusion in ICD–10–AM edition two*. Melbourne, Australia: National Allied Health Casemix Committee.

World Health Organization. (2001). *International classification of functioning, disability and health*. Geneva, Switzerland: Author.

Acquired Brain Injury, Parenting, Social Work, and Rehabilitation: Supporting Parents to Support Their Children

Mark Holloway and Lauren Tyrrell

ABSTRACT

Growing numbers of adults live with the consequences of acquired brain injury (ABI). Those affected frequently require medical input, rehabilitation, and social care. Individuals could suffer from a range of impairments that affect functional abilities. Limited attention has been paid to parenting with an ABI both within the social work and ABI literature. Parents with ABI present specific challenges to social workers and rehabilitationists. Case studies are used to illustrate how services can work to protect and support all parties, facilitating engagement with rehabilitation. The article concludes by considering the knowledge needed to facilitate engagement with rehabilitation and support.

As rates of survival from acquired brain injury (ABI), caused by trauma (traumatic brain injury [TBI]) or otherwise, have improved in both Australia and the United Kingdom (Fortune & Wen, 1999; Headway, 2015a), the numbers of individuals living with the consequences of such injuries increases. The majority of individuals who report to a hospital with a head injury survive and return to the community (National Institute of Clinical Excellence, 2014; Schneider, 2010). International studies have shown that the likelihood of TBI is affected both by gender and socioeconomic status (Hyder, Wunderlich, Puvanachandra, Gururaj, & Kobusingye, 2007), with males and individuals from poorer backgrounds more likely to sustain injury.

Specialist rehabilitation is noted to be effective for ABI (Oddy & Da Silva Ramos, 2013; Turner-Stokes, Disler, Nair, & Wade, 2005), however access to such services is limited particularly in the case of those with mild to moderate injuries, most of whom will be discharged home with no specialist follow-up services (Headway, 2015b).

The behavioral and emotional consequences of ABI, in particular in the context of the impact of reduced insight, can make engagement with rehabilitation services extremely difficult to maintain. Psychosocial functioning is noted to deteriorate over time for some individuals (Holloway, 2012; Medley & Powell, 2010; Ownsworth, McFarland, & Young, 2000; Prigatano, 2005).

A number of individuals who suffer an ABI will either be parents at the time of injury or might become so subsequently; it is inevitable therefore that there will be some intersection with child protection services for some. The nature of the outcome of ABI might well be tested by the challenges of parenting and the impact of this could be felt by the noninjured child (Uysal, Hibbard, Robillard, Pappadopulos, & Jaffe, 1998). Specialist neurorehabilitation services for parents with an ABI are noted to not routinely involve and include children in their work (Webster & Daisley, 2007) despite the benefits of doing so (Edwards, Daisley, & Newby, 2014).

In both Australia and the United Kingdom, it is intended that children are afforded protection from harm by legislation and by child protection or children's safeguarding services that are established accordingly (Council of Australian Governments, 2012; Department for Children, Schools, & Families, 2004; HM Government, 2015; Miller, 2007). Social workers are duty-bound to apply relevant laws, albeit in adult social care, are noted to do so less explicitly than in children's services (Braye, Preston-Shoot, & Wigley, 2013). Such services are generally not aware of ABI or the consequences of the condition (Holloway, 2014) and therefore their input cannot be guided by the functional, emotional, and behavioral consequences of ABI, sometimes with devastating impact for the child, with serious harm caused (Boduszek & Hyland, 2012; Summerfield, 2011). There is, however, recognition of the need to build the knowledge base of social workers in adult settings to provide greater protection for children (Scott, 2009).

The authors of this article note that the sometimes subtle and invisible consequences of ABI can greatly affect an individual (Department of Health, SSI, 1996; Simpson, Simons, & McFadyen, 2002), leading to difficulties with successful community reintegration and functioning. Difficulties with executive impairment and changes to personality and behavior are potentially less straightforward for social workers to assess and respond to than more obvious physical impairment (Bach & David, 2006; Barkley, 2012; Manchester, Priestley, & Jackson, 2004). Loss of insight precludes the person with the ABI from being fully aware of his or her needs and how to respond to them (Flashman & McAllister, 2002), reducing the opportunity for peer support and learning (Prigatano, 1991). Lack of insight into the impact of executive impairment is noted to increase the need for external case management (Clark-Wilson et al., 2016). This article focuses primarily on individuals with an ABI who require support to parent for reasons unrelated to physical impairments.

Both authors of this article have taken a professional interest over a number of years in supporting parenting by people with an ABI. We note in our practice that the challenge of parenting for individuals with an ABI requires a person, condition, and unique family system specific response. Doing so bridges the professional worlds and ontologies of both ABI and child development and protection for the benefit of all. Positively, experience shows that using parents' intrinsic motivation to be the best they can for their child can symbiotically create conditions that promote engagement with rehabilitation and support services and improve parenting ability, aiding both child and parent. Conversely, there are occasions when the nature of the injury and the circumstances created are such as to make safe parenting impossible. ABI-aware social workers, with sufficient knowledge of what works, are well placed to both support engagement with rehabilitation and assess parenting to limit risk of harm to children.

Within this article the different approaches undertaken by the authors are examined via the use of two extended case studies.

Acquired brain injury: The impact on the individual

The consequences of ABI are extremely varied (Engberg & Teasdale, 2004; Lees, 1988; Temkin, Corrigan, Dikmen, & MacHamer, 2009), both in terms of severity of impairment experienced and the functional impact this has on an individual and his or her roles, such as parenting. People with a brain injury are noted to have a worse outcome than those with an orthopedic injury (Dahm & Ponsford, 2015) and to suffer worse quality of life than those with other conditions (Brown & Vandergoot, 1998; Jacobsson, Westerberg, & Lexell, 2010) although conversely, posttraumatic growth has also been reported (Powell, Ekin-Wood, & Collin, 2007).

People with an ABI regularly complain of fatigue (Ponsford, Schönberger, & Rajaratnam, 2015) and are assessed to have a range of cognitive and executive difficulties, including difficulties with memory, attention, planning, reasoning, organizing, initiation and motivation, and mood and behavior (Fleminger & Ponsford, 2005; Powell, 1997). Such changes and difficulties challenge the complex role of parenting considerably. The long-term, multifaceted, and all-encompassing nature of the condition has led to some authors noting the need for ABI to be considered a chronic and lifetime condition rather than a "one-off event" (Masel & Dewitt, 2010).

The impact of these impairments in day-to-day functioning understandably varies, but is noted to negatively affect return to work (McCrimmon & Oddy, 2006; Radford et al., 2013) and relationship status (Wood & Yurdakul, 1997). Emotional dysfunction is noted to cause impairment to behavioral competencies in the community (Anderson, Barrash, Bechara, & Tranel, 2006). Such difficulties have a clear potential impact on parental resources and parenting ability.

Research indicates that individuals with an ABI are overrepresented in both homeless and prison populations (Oddy, Frances-Moir, Fortescue, & Chadwick, 2012; Shiroma, Ferguson, & Pickelsimer, 2012) and that rates of suicide are over three times that of community controls (Simpson & Tate, 2007). Similarly people with an ABI are overrepresented in dual-diagnosis drug and mental health treatment centers and are noted to have more complex and difficult-to-treat conditions (Corrigan, Bogner, & Holloman, 2012; Corrigan & Deutschle, 2008; Fleminger, 2013).

For some, behavior following ABI is noted to be very difficult either in terms of active and negative behaviors such as aggression and violence (Freedman & Hemenway, 2000; Giles & Manchester, 2006; O'Sullivan, Glorney, Sterr, Oddy, & Da Silva Ramos, 2015), or more passive ones such as variability of performance, lack of initiation, and self-neglect (Anderson et al., 2006; Braye, Orr, & Preston-Shoot, 2011; Stuss, Murphy, Binns, & Alexander, 2003). Friendship and social networks are noted to deteriorate for some postinjury (Rowlands, 2000).

The impact of ABI on family functioning is noted to be significant (Ergh, Rapport, Coleman, & Hanks, 2002; Tam, McKay, Sloan, & Ponsford, 2015) and noninjured relatives report feelings of grief (Boss, 1999), often unresolved (Oddy & Herbert, 2003; Perlesz, Kinsella, & Crowe, 1999), leading to "ambiguous loss" (Petersen & Sanders, 2015), where, unlike with a bereavement, the injured party is physically present but psychologically changed.

> When the adjective *ambiguous* is used to describe a loss, it means there is no validation or clarification of the loss, and thus a lack of knowing whether the lost person is irretrievably lost or coming back again (Boss, 2006, p. 144).

Quality of spousal relationships following ABI is noted to deteriorate (Gosling & Oddy, 1999), with the impact of the stress of such situations increasing over time (Levor & Jansen, 2000). Although less commonly discussed in the literature, the impact of ABI on siblings is noted to be considerable (Degeneffe & Lee, 2010; Degeneffe & Olney, 2010). Noninjured family members are noted to have no "road-map" to help them cope with such changes (Jordan & Linden, 2013) and this ambiguity can lead to a lack of clarity that creates conflicting and sometimes contradictory emotions (Boss, 2010; Webb, 1998). In extremes, the reaction of non-brain-injured individuals to the impact of injury to loved ones is noted to be catastrophic (Barnes, 2015).

Despite the potential for social workers, in all fields, to come regularly into contact with people with an ABI, the academic literature underpinning the profession is noted to be scant (Mantell et al., 2012). Social workers in Australia and the United Kingdom have a role in assessing risk (to the individual, family, or wider community) and act as potential gatekeepers to resources that might support community reintegration and participation. It is unclear from the literature how social workers' assessments are informed by specific knowledge of ABI (Holloway & Fyson, 2015).

Acquired brain injury: Rehabilitation

Outside of the field of social work literature, the subject of effective rehabilitation for the consequences of ABI is one subject to a great deal of research. Significant methodological difficulties are acknowledged with regard to assessing the efficacy of rehabilitation, in particular difficulties with achieving randomized control trials, heterogeneity of outcome, and even with ethical concerns undertaking such research (Teasell et al., 2007). The authors of this article contend that the ABI rehabilitation literature is, however, key to the process of social work with parents with an ABI. Understanding the impact of the injury and what works to support positive changes and growth, across a lifetime, is central and integral to the social work task, not peripheral or separate.

Involving the injured party in goal setting is noted to result in significant improvement in goal achievement and, just as important, goal maintenance (Cullen, Chundamala, Bayley, & Jutai, 2007) with a requirement for services to focus on the needs of the individual, not the service provider (Bajo & Fleminger, 2002). Involving uninjured family members is reported to be both required and beneficial for ongoing community rehabilitation (Fisher, Lennon, Bellon, & Lawn, 2015; Pace et al., 1999). Goal attainment is noted to be significantly better in families that function and communicate better with each other (Barclay, 2013) and poorer family functioning is indicated in worse rehabilitation outcomes (Sander et al., 2002).

The use of "real-life" contexts by which to learn from experience in the community is highlighted as effective (Carlson et al., 2006) and rehabilitation is even noted to be effective for those who are slow to recover, often with more profound needs (Gray, 2000).

Creating and sustaining engagement between brain-injured people and rehabilitation and support services is recognized as complex (Medley & Powell, 2010). The consequences of ABI can undermine motivation, act as a barrier to initiation, and prevent individuals from conceptualizing abstract ideas such as goal setting and the steps required for their achievement (Holloway, 2012; Prigatano, 2005, 2008). Adjusting the approach to suit client need is required (Jackson & Chable, 1985). Loss of insight is identified as having a damaging impact on capacity to adhere to treatment (Trahan, Pepin, & Hopps, 2006).

Providing the opportunity for "errorless learning" is noted to be beneficial for some brain-injured people, particularly for those with more severe memory impairment (Baddeley & Wilson, 1994; Clare & Jones, 2008; Evans et al., 2000). Consistency of approach and message is noted to be very important to support effective rehabilitation (Chamberlain, Neumann, & Tennant, 1995; Giles & Clark-Wilson, 1993; Jackson et al., 2014). The removal of ambiguity prevents those with cognitive or executive impairments from picking up mixed messages or being unclear about feedback or expectations.

Where some individuals are noted to be able to benefit from cognitive skills retraining (Rohling, Faust, Beverly, & Demakis, 2009), for others a functional approach to rehabilitation, particularly postacute and in the community, is identified as more effective (Clark-Wilson, Giles, & Baxter, 2014). This approach, intended to be client centered and nonaversive, is considered particularly suitable for those who have reduced insight into their condition and live in the community. It is predicated on a therapeutic alliance and positions the worker therefore "in the world" of the client where relationships are key (Beresford, Croft, & Adshead, 2008; Calhoun & Tedeschi, 2012; Flesaker & Larsen, 2012). As such, the principles behind the approach (real-life, relationship-based, promoting independence while acknowledging constraints) sits within social workers' common practice, enabling the skilled and knowledgeable social worker to act as "expert companion" (Calhoun & Tedeschi, 2006). A good working alliance is noted to be key to rehabilitative work (Schönberger, Humle, & Teasdale, 2006).

This therapeutic alliance is tested by both the impact of the brain injury itself, where relationships are complicated by the interrelated changes to thinking, behavior, and emotion (Morton & Wehman, 1995; Shorland & Douglas, 2010), but also by the role a social worker plays in assessing child safety and parenting ability. This is a test of the skills of the social worker, but one that might be supported by siting the brain-injured person central within the process, looking at strengths (Rowlands, 2001), working to include parents in the process (Appleton, Terlektsi, & Coombes, 2015), and developing a greater understanding of the issues of loss of social identity that ABI brings (Martin, Levack, & Sinnott, 2014). As parenting, for many, is an integral part of social identity, then supporting the restructuring of a new postinjury identity is part of the task that supports parenting itself (Nochi, 2000; Segal, 2010). The act of parenting post ABI has been identified as supporting positive personal growth for the parents concerned (Edwards et al., 2014; Holloway, 2016).

Overall, although methodological difficulties in assessing the effectiveness of neurorehabilitation in its various guises are observed, there is a growing body of evidence that indicates it is worthwhile in terms of both return to independent functioning and reduction in care and support costs (Oddy & Da Silva Ramos, 2013; Turner-Stokes, 2008; Wood, McCrea, Wood, & Merriman, 1999; Worthington, Matthews, Melia, & Oddy, 2006). The role of social work within such research is ill-defined, but social workers (and social-work-trained brain injury case managers) do work with this group both in inpatient and community settings (Carlton & Stephenson, 1990; Clark-Wilson & Holloway, 2015; Lees, 1988; Parker, 2006). Of more relevance perhaps is that the techniques, knowledge, and approaches undertaken by rehabilitation-focused staff need to be understood and applied by all social workers to ensure that their endeavors are based within the needs of the injured party and their family.

There is little in the body of literature, written by social workers, to describe how condition-specific knowledge is applied (Mantell et al., 2012).

Parenting following an ABI: The literature

Parenting, and the responsibilities that come with the role, remain filled with emotions and expectations that can test and challenge the abilities of even the most prepared person. Parenting is characterized by constant change: This needs to be navigated by parents, and although the role might be exciting and considered a privilege, it can also be daunting, exhausting, and anxiety provoking. Usually parents want the best for their children and a variety of supports, informal and formal, will always be needed to augment this (Kolar, Weston, & Soriano, 2001). Additional complexities, such as ABI, require that the support parents receive matches their needs. If risk of significant harm is present, then ethically and legally the necessity to respond is apparent.

Negative impact on parenting and children

The skills and abilities to parent adequately, to provide an environment that nurtures and supports child development, can clearly be challenged by the impact of ABI. Noting the heterogeneous nature of ABI, and indeed of families, the role of parent is one that tests abilities over an extended time frame. The negative impact of parental brain injury on children is recorded in the literature. Injured parents have been recorded as being less nurturing and less involved than their non-brain-injured counterparts (Uysal et al., 1998) with increased risk, for the child, of emotional and behavioral difficulties (Butera-Prinzi & Perlesz, 2004; Pessar, Coad, Linn, & Willer, 1993).

A phenomenological study of children's response to parental brain injury identified key and repeating themes of loss experienced by children, a loss that is often suppressed by the child to protect the injured parent (Kieffer-Kristensen & Johansen, 2013). Children's emotional functioning is also identified to be dependent on the level of stress experienced by the noninjured parent (Kieffer-Kristensen, Siersma, & Teasdale, 2013). The stress of the noninjured partner is noted to be raised as a consequence of the injury, with increased family dysfunction and reduced satisfaction in the relationship (Kieffer-Kristensen & Teasdale, 2011).

There is some evidence that the impact of ABI in the family has a gendered component in relation to the influence of disrupted family functioning on level of distress in males (Anderson, Simpson, & Morey, 2013). A review of the literature on the impact of parental ABI on children highlights the variability of outcome for them but notes the risks and need for such children to have particular attention paid to their needs (Tiar & Dumas, 2015).

Childhood development necessitates that the approach taken to support parents (and their children) changes over time as the child's needs change: "A first step for clinicians to understand is that parents' and families' needs for support will not follow a predictable linear path, and to prepare to adapt their practice flexibly accordingly" (Skippon, 2013, p. 303).

Negative impact on the wider family

Although the brain injury is most usually only directly experienced by one parent, the impact of the injury on a child's other parent, if involved in their upbringing, could have a knock-on impact on the noninjured party's parenting too. As previously noted, the quality of relationships following injury can be deleteriously affected, with increased levels of spousal dissatisfaction, depression, separation, and stress (Blake, 2014; Levor & Jansen, 2000; Simpson & Baguley, 2012; Tam et al., 2015; Winstanley, Simpson, Tate, & Myles, 2006).

Less than adequate parenting increases the risk of exposure to physical, sexual, and emotional abuse; neglect; and family violence. Cumulatively, childhood development can be affected and early intervention remains the best chance to protect children and support families (Higgins & Katz, 2008; Munro, 2011).

The following case studies aim to provide examples of how injured people have been supported to parent in both the United Kingdom (Jane) and Australia (Belle). Table 1 provides a précis of preinjury, injury, postinjury rehabilitation, and community discharge details for both cases.

All names and identifying details have been removed and permission has been sought from both families to create these anonymized case studies.

Case study 1: Bespoke individualized support (UK)

Injury and impact

As outlined in Table 1, Jane sustained her injury at the age of 13. Five years post-discharge, at age 18, Jane suffered from a range of physical, cognitive, executive, behavioral, and emotional difficulties. Jane was a wheelchair user, albeit able to transfer and manage in her home without mobility equipment. She suffered from fatigue and depression, was impulsive and disinhibited, found independent reasoning and abstract thinking difficult, had severe attention deficits and slowed speed of processing, was unable to plan or organize, and lacked much awareness of risk either from environmental dangers (e.g., road crossing) or from people in the environment. Jane suffered from mild dysphagia, but would not use thickeners in her drinks, would regularly fall when she failed to take account of her physical impairments when mobilizing, and would occasionally drink alcohol to excess. Jane regularly suffered from chest infections.

Table 1. Summary of case studies.

	Jane (UK)	Belle (Australia)
Preinjury	Youngest of three siblings in a lone-parent household of poor socioeconomic circumstances. Jane had achieved relatively well at school and had met all of her developmental milestones.	Belle worked as a laboratory assistant (studying applied chemistry) and her husband Dean drove trucks. Belle is the second child of four from a nuclear family.
Injury	Pedestrian victim of road traffic accident at age 13.	At age 25 Belle experienced an acute myocardial infarction resulting in a permanent pacemaker and hypoxia.
Immediate aftermath	Lowest Glasgow Coma Scale (GCS) 4, coma for 18 weeks; posttraumatic amnesia (PTA) of 6 months plus, defined as very severe traumatic brain injury with focal frontal lobe and widespread diffuse axonal injuries.	GCS at the scene was 6/15. Major residual difficulties with fatigue, persistent significant memory disturbance for auditory and verbal information, mild psychomotor slowing and attention difficulties.
Rehabilitation and early care	Jane remained in hospital for duration of coma and was then discharged to a pediatric neurorehabilitation unit. Initially Jane required full nursing care to enable her to eat, wash, and dress.	In 2002 and 2003 Belle had medical and rehabilitation follow-up on discharge from hospital but declined ongoing rehabilitation. Belle's life became further complicated by the emergence of bipolar disorder after several episodes of acute mania. On discharge in 2008 from acute psychiatric services a referral was put into a family services program.
Circumstances at discharge	Jane was discharged after 1 year to the care of her mother. At this stage she could dress and bathe with assistance and could feed herself. Jane was wheelchair reliant, prone to anger outbursts, suffered extreme fatigue, and was emotionally labile. Attempts were made to reintegrate her back into mainstream secondary school. These attempts failed and Jane did not attend school from age 15.	Rehabilitation was requested again in 2011 by her general practitioner, who requested assistance regarding her ability to run the home and parent her children. As a consequence of her brain injury, Belle has impaired memory and suffers from fatigue and severe labile mood. Rehabilitation team remain actively involved.

As the accident to Jane was caused by partial negligence of an insured driver, litigation was undertaken on her behalf and a settlement achieved to contribute toward the cost of support services and for loss of earnings. Jane was defined in UK law as lacking the ability to manage her funds, property, and affairs as a function of her brain injury and a Court of Protection Deputy, a specialist solicitor, was appointed to undertake financial management and decision making on her behalf.

The Deputy commissioned an independent and specialist brain injury case management company to work with Jane and her family to promote her ongoing rehabilitation, to provide her with bespoke support so she could access the community, and to limit the risks she posed to herself and that were posed to her by others.

Jane would frequently ask for support, in particular to enable her to undertake activities away from her home, but did not sustain her interest or agreement for any activity, often dismissing support work staff and refusing to allow them to continue to work with her. A lengthy history was developed regarding Jane engaging and disengaging with services and of her family playing a part in actively undermining her progress and attempts at community-based rehabilitation.

On several occasions, the independent brain injury case manager referred to statutory social work colleagues to carry out investigations into alleged abuse of Jane by family owing to issues with Jane's resources being taken advantage of and with aggression in the household aimed at Jane. Although Jane did receive support throughout this period, it was more ad hoc and reactive to difficulties rather than a planned and structured intervention as the situation within the house was, on occasion, extremely chaotic.

Jane in a relationship

Approximately 10 years postinjury, Jane met and married Peter, a long-term user of mental health services for reasons of enduring depression; he had attempted suicide on several occasions. Peter moved into the home with Jane and her mother. Peter was very motivated to work, but found it difficult to maintain employment owing to his low mood. The nature of the relationship between Peter and Jane's mother was one marked by regular arguments and aggression, leading to the police being called on several occasions.

Jane voluntarily contacted her brain injury case manager to inform him of her decision to start a family. Both of Jane's siblings and her mother had, at various points, been involved with statutory social workers as concerns had been raised regarding their parenting abilities. Jane was aware that her ability to parent would be questioned and agreed that her case manager should contact the relevant authorities to discuss this when she became pregnant, as she did in due course.

Initial response of statutory services

Early indication from the social work team was that an order would be sought through the UK courts to remove Jane's child at birth. After discussion with the team it became clear that this decision was predicated on factors that related to Jane but also to others in her milieu. Overall, Jane was not able or willing to recognize the impact that parenting would have on her compromised abilities or vice-versa, and furthermore, lacked insight into her difficulties, often only being able to see problems in hindsight and being unable to learn easily from this process. Furthermore, Peter and Jane wanted Jane's mother to leave the family home, but were unable to address this with her.

Table 2. Intervention to support parenting.

Injury and psychosocial challenges	Potential impact on child's well-being
Jane's functional status	
Jane was not able to assess risk, frequently falling despite acknowledging her physical impairments Failed to follow advice regarding her swallowing difficulties Lacked a sense of road safety	Might injure herself and not be able to tend to the baby Might not appropriately judge activities that could expose baby to risk of harm
Jane's physical impairments would preclude her from carrying a baby safely but she had issues with impulsivity and insight	Likely to carry out such actions despite the risk of injury to the baby if she did fall
Cognitive and executive difficulties were such that she was unable to independently plan and structure her time and was not able to eat regularly or take medication to prescription	Unable to care adequately for her own basic needs Unable to structure adequate care routine for baby Unable to identify and respond to ill health or risk
Lengthy history of not maintaining engagement with support services, frequently disengaging at points of perceived confrontation, difficulty, or low mood	Staffing essential to support Jane to parent not possible to maintain, leading to frequent and destabilizing changes and undue risk
Jane's broader psychosocial context	
Peter had significant mental health problems that were exacerbated by stress	Unable to support Jane to change her view or behavior; challenges in playing the parent role himself
Jane's mother remained in the home with Peter and Jane	Openly hostile to the statutory social work team and unlikely to accept the presence of the intensive staffing support that Jane would require coming into the house

The specific concerns identified by the social workers are summarized in Table 2.

Intervention to support parenting.

Following negotiation with the statutory social work team, the case manager, working with others, coordinated the following intervention to support Jane to parent:

- An interdisciplinary team (IDT) was created consisting of the case manager, a neuropsychologist, a specialist health visitor, and three support workers.
- It was agreed that, initially, a support worker would always need to be present when Jane was alone with her daughter, Lisa.
- It was agreed that only the health visitor would provide advice and instruction or guidance with regard to parenting and that the other IDT members would defer to her at all times to prevent Jane from receiving accidentally mixed messages.
- The IDT met regularly to exchange information, monitor progress and challenges, and adapt advice and instruction for the support workers as Lisa developed and her needs and presentation changed.

- The health visitor provided advice and guidance regarding likely upcoming developmental changes that would require planning and intervention.
- The neuropsychologist held regular meetings with Jane and Peter to identify how they were coping, provide strategies to support parenting, provide positive reinforcement concerning their successful parenting, and support changes that were upcoming in line with the health visitor's predictions of Lisa's likely development.
- As a consequence of the neuropsychologist's input, Jane was able to be supported to understand that her mood and functioning were negatively affected by her fatigue and she began to regularly rest during the day. This had a significant impact.
- The neuropsychologist provided specific instructions and advice to the support work team regarding the wholly consistent approach that was required to support Jane to succeed. Specific scripts and phrases were developed to prevent ambiguity. Jane was supported to parent; the staff did not undertake a parenting role on her behalf.
- The case manager provided regular face-to-face supervision of the support work staff. Initially contact with the support work team was daily via text messages, e-mail, and telephone calls.
- The support workers completed an agreed e-mail-based daily recording sheet. The health visitor, neuropsychologist, and case manager designed the recording sheet to ensure that this elicited the information that was required to monitor risk and changes to Lisa as she developed. This recording sheet was sent to every member of the IDT each day.
- The support workers' guide and risk assessment documents were reviewed regularly in light of changes that were encountered as Lisa developed. Each member of the IDT was involved in these changes with the support workers playing an active role.
- Following a deterioration in the relationship between Jane and her mother, the case manager sought and sourced alternative social housing provision for Jane's mother and facilitated her leaving Jane's home.
- Prior to Lisa being able to independently communicate clearly, Jane was unable to identify when her daughter was unwell and act appropriately, necessitating staff intervention. The IDT had predicted the likelihood of Jane's lack of capacity to act in her daughter's best interests in this event and all documentation instructed staff of their responsibility to act unilaterally to refer to medical staff. This included a required hospital admission on one occasion. Jane was able to understand this in hindsight only.
- Lisa has been supported directly and indirectly by the IDT to learn and understand her mother's brain injury by the provision of age-appropriate literature and the development of agreed "scripts" that support workers and Jane use to explain what her brain injury means and normalize this accordingly.

Outcome

- Jane has been supported to parent successfully for more than 8 years.
- During this time, there has been one change of support work staff (after 6 years, departure of staff for personal reasons) and Lisa has met and exceeded all age-related milestones.
- Lisa is academically able and is noted by school staff to have better social abilities than many peers. Lisa has a friendship circle and regularly attends after-school activities and groups.
- There have been no instances where Jane has wholly refused to accept the advice of her clinical team, but there has been one instance where achieving her agreement took a concerted intervention. This occurred when Jane wished to have an extended period of informal family support instead of paid provision.
- Jane rests and prepares meals on a daily basis, undertakes voluntary work at a school, initiates planning sessions with her support workers, has not had a reoccurrence of her depression, regularly attends meetings with her IDT, and is both more structured and engaged with her team.
- Jane remains unable to predict likely changes to Lisa and her behavior as she ages, requiring the IDT, to a lesser extent than previously, to maintain a role of preempting difficulties and supporting changes and novel problem solving. Hours of support work have reduced by 33% and case management and neuropsychology by over 66% each. This reduction in input has been slow, structured, and monitored. Jane now spends agreed time with Lisa without a member of support staff being present.

The initially enforced structure and support provided to Jane has facilitated her development toward rehabilitation goals and functional independence that she previously had been unable to agree to or, if able to agree to, been unable to sustain. Jane's contact with her case manager is no longer as reactive and crisis-driven. The improvements to her functioning (including her parenting) are a consequence of her engagement with her IDT and, from a brain injury rehabilitation perspective, are interesting as they did not take place until Jane was more than 12 years postinjury. Jane voluntarily and happily engages with her team, seeing the value they add to her life. Parenting is a goal that Jane intrinsically believed to be valuable. Peter has maintained better mental health and has consistently been in full-time work for more than 5 years.

Case study 2: Specialist rehabilitation service (Australia)

Injury and impact

Belle and Dean attended postacute treatment with a trauma rehabilitation team with goals to develop strategies around her daily living and to return to work as a laboratory assistant. Unable to return to her former job and advised medically against having children, Belle withdrew from rehabilitation.

Ten years postinjury, the rehabilitation medical consultant requested social work follow-up with the family and phone contact was made with Dean. They had moved to a rural area; Belle was working at a chicken farm and they had two children, Zoe, 7 years old at the time, and Harry, 5 years old, and had limited family support. Dean spoke about isolation within their community and shared an experience. "We went to Carols by Candlelight. We put our picnic blanket down like everyone else, but no one sat next to us, no one spoke to us." Dean was initially ambivalent about rehabilitation involvement. The first stage was engagement and developing a relationship, acknowledging and honoring his hopes and expectations, working at his pace.

Belle had low tolerance of her children's behavior, becoming agitated easily and regularly shouting at them, particularly when having to multitask, such as at meal times. When home, Dean saw himself as the mediator. The stress of the household was evident as problems at home and school were apparent in the children's behavior: Zoe with encopresis, Harry with anger outbursts, and both children noted to be socially isolated at school.

Belle in a relationship

It was observed that Dean put the rules in place, sometimes undermining Belle's decisions in situations he felt were too strict. Belle accepted his direction, but reported feeling undermined. Harry, in particular, would become disrespectful toward Belle and arguments would ensue. Belle was dismissive of Zoe if she felt she was excessively seeking her attention. Dean resorted to drinking alcohol and smoking marijuana in the evenings. Belle would drink, too.

Dean recognized the family behavioral patterns, but still hoped that Belle could manage and things would get better. At times he would normalize their behaviors, suggesting all families had issues. One of Dean's sisters, a teacher, offered some support regarding Zoe's encopresis, but this served to affirm Dean and Belle's beliefs that Zoe was attention seeking and manipulative.

Initial response of statutory services

Over time, Dean was able to provide more information regarding the family's functioning. A child protection notification had been made when Zoe, as a baby, fell from a changing table, breaking her collarbone, but there was no further service input.

When both children were of preschool age, Belle had an acute mental health episode resulting in a diagnosis of and treatment for bipolar disorder. On discharge, a family services program was referred to for support and monitoring.

Intervention to support parenting

The family services and rehabilitation social workers collaborated to support the family collaboratively achieving the following strategies:

- Belle started seeing the rehabilitation clinical psychologist. Psychoeducation was provided to Dean regarding the severity of Belle's brain injury with the combined impact of bipolar disorder and her preaccident functioning and beliefs regarding parenting. Some changes in clinical psychology staffing affected Belle's commitment to participate for a time until her primary psychologist returned. Over time Belle could state "my high expectations of the kids have changed."
- As money was a pressure for Dean and Belle, and a potential barrier to participating, the rehabilitation social worker applied for fee waiver of service.
- The rehabilitation social worker supported Dean and Belle at regular school meetings. A psychologist from the education department became involved to support behavioral management strategies for the teachers regarding the children's respective behaviors.
- Both social workers encouraged Dean to see his general practitioner (GP) about a mental health plan for Zoe and Harry, resulting in a private psychologist working with the children.
- Social work accessed secondary consultation with the ABI team, resulting in implementation of behavioral modification strategies with Zoe such as star charts and rewards, an accepted first-stage treatment option for fecal encopresis. Dean and Belle maintained they had already tried all strategies without success, and their doubtful view marred the potential success of the follow-on phase of narrative work.
- With Dean's consent, the family services social worker engaged the GP, who reviewed Zoe's medical situation, resulting in medication and hospital input.
- Dean admitted to being depressed, but declined seeing his GP; however, the rehabilitation social worker maintained contact, encouraging him to seek treatment.
- The family services social worker left and the family did not wish to engage someone new. Referral back to family services resulted in the family being assessed as improved and coping, and therefore low priority. Without a worker present in the home to monitor, the rehabilitation social worker continues as the primary contact, maintaining engagement with Dean, although less able to undertake frequent home visits.
- Acknowledging the family's isolation, the rehabilitation social worker ran the ABI Family to Family Link Up program.
- Four family sessions cofacilitated by the rehabilitation social worker and the private psychologist were attended but terminated due to the session times disrupting family meal routines. One outcome was an agreement

to provide psychoeducation to Zoe only, with Dean feeling that Harry was too young to involve.

Outcome

Dean has recently seen his GP and started medication regarding his alcohol addiction and the rehabilitation social worker will continue to maintain engagement with him and Belle using a drug and alcohol harm minimization approach. The rehabilitation team social worker and clinical psychologist will develop a process for future therapeutic family work, inclusive of the children and significant extended family members, aiming to provide psychoeducation to them regarding Belle's brain injury, then structure both one-on-one and couple work toward addressing the stress in the family. Future work for the children will require closer and more transparent practice between the rehabilitation team, private psychologist, and teachers, with regular correspondence to the GP.

Dean's commitment remains pivotal to much of the work and the balance of his emotional needs will continue to be monitored. Small achievable goals that can be reviewed and measured regularly have been developed with Belle and Dean. The service aims are to reduce stress and therefore symptomatic behaviors, remove internal family blame and shame that is so often experienced by families living with ABI, and work toward strategies for managing on a day-to-day basis. Interventions provided by a range of services require transparent complementary practice and clear communication.

Although rehabilitation is not funded for case management, continuity of the key worker is essential for this family and the rehabilitation team has made a commitment to the long-term support required for this complex work. Secondary consultation with the ABI team will continue as therapeutic advice and resources are shared. The external perspective can highlight service risks such as compassion fatigue and over- or underservicing. Additionally, continuity of services and staff also prevents further rejection, as with the aforementioned community experience. The rehabilitation social worker continues to coordinate the service response to Belle and her family. With the risk of the family falling through service gaps or potentially receiving further tertiary service responses, the ABI rehabilitation services bring the perspective and vigilance needed to work with this family to prevent such occurrences and support the broader goal of health and well-being.

Lessons learned from the case studies

The approach taken in the United Kingdom and Australia has facilitated engagement (Medley & Powell, 2010), has recognized the specific risks to children as a consequence of parental brain injury (Tiar & Dumas, 2015), and has strengthened family functioning (Appleton et al., 2015), predicting and reacting to family need (Skippon, 2013).

For social workers engaged in the field of child safeguarding, the lessons are those of needing to fully understand the impact of an injury that causes changes to parenting and to understand the approaches that work and support change following an ABI. The key message for social workers is that the nature of ABI requires a proactive approach to engage and support families and not simply a reactive, crisis-driven, and safeguarding-led one.

Discussion

As can be seen by the case studies provided, the unique nature of both families requires a highly individualized response, a bespoke intervention in the case of the UK example, and a highly specialized and dedicated service in the Australian case. Despite the uniqueness of each family and cross-border cultural and legal differences, commonality is found with regard to social work practice, including the social workers' imperative to protect children according to relevant legislation.

Social workers in both case studies have needed to use the skills, knowledge, and experience of other professional staff across varying disciplines. They have needed to understand and respond to the specific functional ABI-related difficulties of the individual with whom they are working. In addition, it has been important to incorporate an understanding of child development within the response provided to families and a need to work within (and on occasion on) the social milieu of the family, viewing the family as a "system" and not disparate individuals.

Social workers working with parents with an ABI need to appeal to the intrinsic motivation of the injured parent and other family members to maximize the impact of the intervention provided. The need to practice social work in a proactive way over lengthy time periods, predicting difficulties and supporting a response to them in advance of harm, not as a response to harm already caused, is also key to effective work in this complex setting.

The demonstrated approach undertaken both in Australia and in the United Kingdom is informed by practice and research from both inside and outside of the social work literature. Working practically and functionally (Clark-Wilson et al., 2014) with injured people to improve the likelihood first of engagement (Medley & Powell, 2010), and second of improved goal achievement (Cullen et al., 2007), the brain-injury-aware social worker can play a central role in the promotion of effective use of rehabilitation and support by the injured party, monitor risk, and reduce likelihood of harm. By doing so, children and their families are more likely to remain together. This requires an understanding of the impact of ABI, of services that can promote engagement and rehabilitation, and of child development. Supporting children directly, via use of narrative tools and appropriate literature, enables them to give voice to their experience, creating greater understanding of their perceptions by the parents and professionals involved (Butera-Prinzi, Charles, & Story, 2014; Johnson & Densham, 2011), integrating child, family, and rehabilitative needs.

Conclusion

Parenting with or without a brain injury is a difficult role but one that is often the most highly valued by individuals. The nature of ABI with its complex, interrelated, and often invisible sequelae is one that provides truly significant challenges for parents who are affected. By understanding in detail the functional and emotional impact of such injuries (what works to support sustained engagement, rehabilitation, and adaptation), as well as the children's needs over the course of their development, social workers are able to work alongside injured people to appeal to intrinsic motivation to support not only parenting, but also the parents in their own lifetime process of change and adaptation. In doing so, the social worker can act to support the re-creation of a new narrative for an individual, standing as the "expert companion" as a new social identity is crafted (Calhoun & Tedeschi, 2006; Nochi, 2000).

Such input has the potential to have value and impact over the course of generations and is based within the ethical belief system and values that inform our profession and practice as social workers (Baker, Tandy, & Dixon, 2002). By integrating the knowledge of other professionals, we are better equipped to help prevent abuse, accidental or otherwise.

The alternative is to not integrate knowledge of the impact of ABI, of the needs of children as they develop, and of the input that can be provided to support parenting. Doing so places injured parents, the great majority of whom are motivated to do their best, in the invidious position of not being able to request or receive the necessary services that help compensate for complex interrelated impairments, increasing risk of harm or unnecessary intervention that might separate families. Evidence exists of how ABI affects more than the individual concerned within a family, therefore our response needs to do so also (Gan, Campbell, Gemeinhardt, & McFadden, 2006). Supporting family members who support the injured party forms a part of the rehabilitation and well-being of that injured party (Lehan, Arango-Lasprilla, De Los Reyes, & Quijano, 2012).

We argue therefore that ABI and the impact this has on parenting is a red flag for services, both those concerned with child welfare and those concerned with rehabilitation, to work together to achieve better outcomes. The challenge for social workers is to increase their knowledge base, to work alongside others, including family, in partnership, and to view their role as one that develops and changes over time. How can we do this? Bearing in mind what is at stake when considering parenting following a brain injury, perhaps we simply need to follow practical and sage advice, "Do whatever it takes" (Willer & Corrigan, 1994).

Acknowledgments

We would like to thank Dr. Allison Rowlands for her significant support in the preparation of this article and also Jo Clark Wilson and Grahame Simpson for their guidance.

References

Anderson, M. I., Simpson, G. K., & Morey, P. J. (2013). The impact of neurobehavioral impairment on family functioning and the psychological well-being of male versus female caregivers of relatives with severe traumatic brain injury: Multigroup analysis. *Journal of Head Trauma Rehabilitation, 28,* 453–463. doi:10.1097/htr.0b013e31825d6087

Anderson, S. W., Barrash, J., Bechara, A., & Tranel, D. (2006). Impairments of emotion and real-world complex behavior following childhood- or adult-onset damage to ventromedial prefrontal cortex. *Journal of the International Neuropsychological Society, 12,* 224–235. doi:10.1017/s1355617706060346

Appleton, J. V., Terlektsi, E., & Coombes, L. (2015). Implementing the strengthening families approach to child protection conferences. *British Journal of Social Work, 45,* 1395–1414. doi:10.1093/bjsw/bct211

Bach, L. J., & David, A. S. (2006). Self-awareness after acquired and traumatic brain injury. *Neuropsychological Rehabilitation, 16,* 397–414. doi:10.1080/09602010500412830

Baddeley, A., & Wilson, B. A. (1994). When implicit learning fails: Amnesia and the problem of error elimination. *Neuropsychologia, 32,* 53–68. doi:10.1016/0028-3932(94)90068-x

Bajo, A., & Fleminger, S. (2002). Brain injury rehabilitation: What works for whom and when? *Brain Injury, 16,* 385–395. doi:10.1080/02699050110119826

Baker, K. A., Tandy, C. C., & Dixon, D. R. (2002). Traumatic brain injury. *Journal of Social Work in Disability & Rehabilitation, 1,* 25–44.

Barclay, D. A. (2013). Family functioning, psychosocial stress, and goal attainment in brain injury rehabilitation. *Journal of Social Work in Disability and Rehabilitation, 12*, 159–175. doi:10.1080/1536710x.2013.810093

Barkley, R. A. (2012). *Executive functions: What they are, how they work, and why they evolved.* New York, NY: Guilford.

Barnes, M. (2015). *Findings of the inquest into the deaths of the Hunt family.* Wagga Wagga, Australia: State Coroner's Court of New South Wales.

Beresford, P., Croft, S., & Adshead, L. (2008). "We don't see her as a social worker": A service user case study of the importance of the social worker's relationship and humanity. *British Journal of Social Work, 38*, 1388–1407. doi:10.1093/bjsw/bcm043

Blake, H. (2014). Caregiver stress in traumatic brain injury. *International Journal of Therapy and Rehabilitation, 15*, 263–271. doi:10.12968/ijtr.2008.15.6.29878

Boduszek, D., & Hyland, P. (2012). Fred West: Bio-psycho-social investigation of psychopathic sexual serial killer. *International Journal of Criminology and Sociological Theory, 5*, 864–870.

Boss, P. (1999). *Ambiguous loss: Learning to live with unresolved grief.* Cambridge, MA: Harvard University Press.

Boss, P. (2006). *Loss, trauma, and resilience: Therapeutic work with ambiguous loss.* New York, NY: Norton.

Boss, P. (2010). The trauma and complicated grief of ambiguous loss. *Pastoral Psychology, 59*, 137–145. doi:10.1007/s11089-009-0264-0

Braye, S., Orr, D., & Preston-Shoot, M. (2011). Conceptualising and responding to self-neglect: The challenges for adult safeguarding. *Journal of Adult Protection, 13*, 182–193. doi:10.1108/14668201111177905

Braye, S., Preston-Shoot, M., & Wigley, V. (2013). Deciding to use the law in social work practice. *Journal of Social Work, 13*, 75–95. doi:10.1177/1468017311431476v

Brown, M., & Vandergoot, D. (1998). Quality of life for individuals with traumatic brain injury: Comparison with others living in the community. *Journal of Head Trauma Rehabilitation, 13*, 1–23. doi:10.1097/00001199-199808000-00002

Butera-Prinzi, F., Charles, N., & Story, K. (2014). Narrative family therapy and group work for families living with acquired brain injury. *Australian and New Zealand Journal of Family Therapy, 35*, 81–99. doi:10.1002/anzf.1046

Butera-Prinzi, F., & Perlesz, A. (2004). Through children's eyes: Children's experience of living with a parent with an acquired brain injury. *Brain Injury, 18*, 83–101. doi:10.1080/0269905031000118500

Calhoun, L., & Tedeschi, R. (2006). *Expert companions: Posttraumatic growth in clinical practice. Handbook of posttraumatic growth: Research and practice.* Mahwah, NJ: Erlbaum.

Calhoun, L. G., & Tedeschi, R. G. (2012). *Posttraumatic growth in clinical practice.* New York, NY: Taylor & Francis.

Carlson, P. M., Boudreau, M. L., Davis, J., Johnston, J., Lemsky, C., McColl, M. A., … Smith, C. (2006). "Participate to learn": A promising practice for community ABI rehabilitation. *Brain Injury, 20*, 1111–1117. doi:10.1080/02699050600955337

Carlton, T. O., & Stephenson, M. D. G. (1990). Social work and the management of severe head injury. *Social Science and Medicine, 31*, 5–11. doi:10.1016/0277-9536(90)90003-b

Chamberlain, M. A., Neumann, V., & Tennant, A. (1995). *Traumatic brain injury rehabilitation: Services, treatments and outcomes.* London, UK: Chapman & Hall Medical.

Clare, L., & Jones, R. S. P. (2008). Errorless learning in the rehabilitation of memory impairment: A critical review. *Neuropsychology Review, 18*, 1–23. doi:10.1007/s11065-008-9051-4

Clark-Wilson, J., Giles, G. M., & Baxter, D. M. 2014. Revisiting the neurofunctional approach: Conceptualizing the core components for the rehabilitation of everyday living skills. *Brain Injury, 28*, 1646–1656.

Clark-Wilson, J., Giles, G. M., Seymour, S., Tasker, R., Baxter, D. M., & Holloway, M. (2016). Factors influencing community case management and care hours for clients with traumatic brain injury living in the UK. *Brain Injury*, 30, 872–882. doi:10.3109/02699052.2016.1146799

Clark-Wilson, J., & Holloway, M. (2015). Life care planning and long-term care for individuals with brain injury in the UK. *NeuroRehabilitation*, 36, 289–300. doi:10.3233/nre-151217

Corrigan, J. D., Bogner, J., & Holloman, C. (2012). Lifetime history of traumatic brain injury among persons with substance use disorders. *Brain Injury*, 26, 139–150. doi:10.3109/02699052.2011.648705

Corrigan, J. D., & Deutschle, J. J. (2008). The presence and impact of traumatic brain injury among clients in treatment for co-occurring mental illness and substance abuse. *Brain Injury*, 22, 223–231. doi:10.1080/02699050801938967

Council of Australian Governments. (2012). *Protecting children is everyone's business: National framework for protecting Australia's children. Second three-year action plan 2012–2015.* Canberra, Australia: Author.

Cullen, N., Chundamala, J., Bayley, M., & Jutai, J. (2007). The efficacy of acquired brain injury rehabilitation. *Brain Injury*, 21, 113–132. doi:10.1080/02699050701201540

Dahm, J., & Ponsford, J. (2015). Comparison of long-term outcomes following traumatic injury: What is the unique experience for those with brain injury compared with orthopaedic injury? *Injury*, 46, 142–149. doi:10.1016/j.injury.2014.07.012

DeGeneffe, C. E., & Lee, G. K. (2010). Quality of life after traumatic brain injury: Perspectives of adult siblings. *Journal of Rehabilitation*, 76, 27–36.

DeGeneffe, C. E., & Olney, M. F. (2010). "We are the forgotten victims": Perspectives of adult siblings of persons with traumatic brain injury. *Brain Injury*, 24, 1416–1427. doi:10.3109/02699052.2010.514317

Department for Children, Schools, & Families. (2004). *Children act, Great Britain.* Retrieved from http://www.legislation.gov.uk/ukpga/2004/31/contents

Department of Health, SSI. (1996). *A hidden disability: Report of the SSI traumatic brain injury rehabilitation project.* London, UK: Author.

Edwards, A. R., Daisley, A., & Newby, G. (2014). The experience of being a parent with an acquired brain injury (ABI) as an inpatient at a neuro-rehabilitation centre, 0–2 years post-injury. *Brain Injury*, 28, 1700–1710. doi:10.3109/02699052.2014.947633

Engberg, A. W., & Teasdale, T. W. (2004). Psychological outcome following traumatic brain injury in adults: A long term population-based follow-up. *Brain Injury*, 18, 533–545. doi:10.1080/02699050310001645829

Ergh, T. C., Rapport, L. J., Coleman, R. D., & Hanks, R. A. (2002). Predictors of caregiver and family functioning following traumatic brain injury: Social support moderates caregiver distress. *Journal of Head Trauma Rehabilitation*, 17, 155–174. doi:10.1097/00001199-200204000-00006

Evans, J. J., Wilson, B. A., Schuri, U., Andrade, J., Baddeley, A., Bruna, O., ... Taussik, I. (2000). A comparison of "errorless" and "trial-and-error" learning methods for teaching individuals with acquired memory deficits. *Neuropsychological Rehabilitation*, 10, 67–101. doi:10.1080/096020100389309

Fisher, A., Lennon, S., Bellon, M., & Lawn, S. (2015). Family involvement in behaviour management following acquired brain injury (ABI) in community settings: A systematic review. *Brain Injury*, 29, 661–675. doi:10.3109/02699052.2015.1004751

Flashman, L. A., & McAllister, T. W. (2002). Lack of awareness and its impact in traumatic brain injury. *NeuroRehabilitation*, 17, 285–296.

Fleminger, S. (2013). Mental health is central to good neurorehabilitation after TBI. *Brain Impairment*, 14, 2–4. doi:10.1017/brimp.2013.14

Fleminger, S., & Ponsford, J. (2005). Long term outcome after traumatic brain injury. *British Medical Journal, 331*, 1419–1420. doi:10.1136/bmj.331.7530.1419

Flesaker, K., & Larsen, D. (2012). To offer hope you must have hope: Accounts of hope for reintegration counsellors working with women on parole and probation. *Qualitative Social Work, 11*, 61–79. doi:10.1177/1473325010382325

Fortune, N., & Wen, X. (1999). *The definition, incidence and prevalence of acquired brain injury in Australia*. Canberra, Australia: Australian Institute of Health and Welfare.

Freedman, D., & Hemenway, D. (2000). Precursors of lethal violence: A death row sample. *Social Science and Medicine, 50*, 1757–1770. doi:10.1016/s0277-9536(99)00417-7

Gan, C., Campbell, K. A., Gemeinhardt, M., & McFadden, G. T. (2006). Predictors of family system functioning after brain injury. *Brain Injury, 20*, 587–600. doi:10.1080/02699050600743725

Giles, G. M., & Clark-Wilson, J. (1993). *Brain injury rehabilitation: A neurofunctional approach*. London, UK: Chapman & Hall.

Giles, G. M., & Manchester, D. (2006). Two approaches to behavior disorder after traumatic brain injury. *Journal of Head Trauma Rehabilitation, 21*, 168–178. doi:10.1097/00001199-200603000-00009

Gosling, J., & Oddy, M. (1999). Rearranged marriages: Marital relationships after head injury. *Brain Injury, 13*, 785–796. doi:10.1080/026990599121179

Gray, D. S. (2000). Slow-to-recover severe traumatic brain injury: A review of outcomes and rehabilitation effectiveness. *Brain Injury, 14*, 1003–1014. doi:10.1080/02699050050191940

Headway. (2015a). *Brain injury statistics*. Nottingham, UK: Author. Retrieved from https://www.headway.org.uk/brain-injury-statistics.aspx

Headway. (2015b). *Don't cut me out*. Nottingham, UK: Author. Retrieved from https://www.headway.org.uk/get-involved/campaigns/dont-cut-me-out/

Higgins, D., & Katz, I. (2008). Enhancing service systems for protecting children: Promoting child wellbeing and child protection reform in Australia. *Family Matters, 80*, 43–50.

HM Government. (2015). *Working together to safeguard children: Department for Children*. London, UK: Her Majesty's Stationary Office.

Holloway, M. (2012). Motivational interviewing and acquired brain injury. *Social Care and Neurodisability, 3*, 122–130. doi:10.1108/20420911211268740

Holloway, M. (2014). How is ABI assessed and responded to in non-specialist settings? Is specialist education required for all social care professionals? *Social Care and Neurodisability, 5*, 201–213. doi:10.1108/scn-12-2013-0043

Holloway, M. (2016, March). *Parenting post-ABI: Fostering engagement with services 14 years post-injury: A case study*. Paper presented at the International Brain Injury Association's Eleventh World Congress on Brain Injury, The Hague, Netherlands.

Holloway, M., & Fyson, R. (2015). Acquired brain injury, social work and the challenges of personalisation. *British Journal of Social Work, 46*, 1301–1317. doi:10.1093/bjsw/bcv039

Hyder, A. A., Wunderlich, C. A., Puvanachandra, P., Gururaj, G., & Kobusingye, O. C. (2007). The impact of traumatic brain injuries: A global perspective. *NeuroRehabilitation, 22*, 341–353.

Jackson, H. F., Hague, G., Daniels, L., Aguilar, R., Jr., Carr, D., & Kenyon, W. (2014). Structure to self-structuring: Infrastructures and processes in neurobehavioural rehabilitation. *NeuroRehabilitation, 34*, 681–694.

Jackson, S., & Chable, D. (1985). Engagement: A critical aspect of family therapy practice. *Australian and New Zealand Journal of Family Therapy, 6*, 65–69. doi:10.1002/j.1467-8438.1985.tb01116.x

Jacobsson, L. J., Westerberg, M., & Lexell, J. (2010). Health-related quality-of-life and life satisfaction 6–15 years after traumatic brain injuries in northern Sweden. *Brain Injury, 24*, 1075–1086. doi:10.3109/02699052.2010.494590

Johnson, J., & Densham, L. (2011). *"My parent has a brain injury": A guide for young people.* Littlehampton, UK: RWP Group.

Jordan, J., & Linden, M. A. (2013). "It's like a problem that doesn't exist": The emotional well-being of mothers caring for a child with brain injury. *Brain Injury, 27*, 1063–1072. doi:10.3109/02699052.2013.794962

Kieffer-Kristensen, R., & Johansen, K. L. G. (2013). Hidden loss: A qualitative explorative study of children living with a parent with acquired brain injury. *Brain Injury, 27*, 1562–1569. doi:10.3109/02699052.2013.841995

Kieffer-Kristensen, R., Siersma, V. D., & Teasdale, T. W. (2013). Family matters: Parental-acquired brain injury and child functioning. *NeuroRehabilitation, 32*, 59–68.

Kieffer-Kristensen, R., & Teasdale, T. W. (2011). Parental stress and marital relationships among patients with brain injury and their spouses. *NeuroRehabilitation, 28*, 321–330.

Kolar, V., Weston, R., & Soriano, G. (2001). Meeting the challenges of parenting: Factors that enhance and hinder the role of parents. *Family Matters, 58*, 38–45.

Lees, M. (1988). The social and emotional consequences of severe brain injury: The social work perspective. In I. Fussey & G. Giles (Eds.), *Rehabilitation of the severely brain-injured adult: A practical approach*, (pp. 241–261). London, UK: Croom Helm.

Lehan, T., Arango-Lasprilla, J. C., De Los Reyes, C. J., & Quijano, M. C. (2012). The ties that bind: The relationship between caregiver burden and the neuropsychological functioning of TBI survivors. *NeuroRehabilitation, 30*, 87–95.

Levor, K. D., & Jansen, P. (2000). The traumatic onset of disabling injury in a marriage partner: Self-reports of the experience by able-bodied spouses. *Social Work, 36*, 193–201.

Manchester, D., Priestley, N., & Jackson, H. (2004). The assessment of executive functions: Coming out of the office. *Brain Injury, 18*, 1067–1081. doi:10.1080/02699050410001672387

Mantell, A., Simpson, G., Jones, K., Strandberg, T., Simonson, P., & Vungkhanching, M. (2012). Social work practice with traumatic brain injury: The results of a structured review. *Brain Injury, 26*, 459–460.

Martin, R., Levack, W. M. M., & Sinnott, K. A. (2014). Life goals and social identity in people with severe acquired brain injury: An interpretative phenomenological analysis. *Disability and Rehabilitation, 37*, 1234–1241. doi:10.3109/09638288.2014.961653

Masel, B. E., & Dewitt, D. S. (2010). Traumatic brain injury: A disease process, not an event. *Journal of Neurotrauma, 27*, 1529–1540. doi:10.1089/neu.2010.1358

McCrimmon, S., & Oddy, M. (2006). Return to work following moderate-to-severe traumatic brain injury. *Brain Injury, 20*, 1037–1046. doi:10.1080/02699050600909656

Medley, A. R., & Powell, T. (2010). Motivational interviewing to promote self-awareness and engagement in rehabilitation following acquired brain injury: A conceptual review. *Neuropsychological Rehabilitation, 20*, 481–508. doi:10.1080/09602010903529610

Miller, R. M. (2007). *Best interests principles: A conceptual overview.* Department of Human Services (AUS). Retrieved from http://www.dhs.vic.gov.au/__data/assets/pdf_file/0006/449214/the-best-interest-principles-a-conceptual-overview.pdf

Morton, M. V., & Wehman, P. (1995). Psychosocial and emotional sequelae of individuals with traumatic brain injury: A literature review and recommendations. *Brain Injury, 9*, 81–92. doi:10.3109/02699059509004574

Munro, E. (2011). *The Munro review of child protection: Final report: A child-centred system.* Norwich, UK: Department for Education.

National Institute of Clinical Excellence. (2014). *Head injury: Triage, assessment, investigation and early management of head injury in children, young people and adults.* Retrieved from https://www.nice.org.uk/guidance/CG176

Nochi, M. (2000). Reconstructing self-narratives in coping with traumatic brain injury. *Social Science and Medicine, 51*, 1795–1804. doi:10.1016/s0277-9536(00)00111-8

Oddy, M., & Da Silva Ramos, S. (2013). The clinical and cost-benefits of investing in neuro-behavioural rehabilitation: A multi-centre study. *Brain Injury, 27,* 1500–1507. doi:10.3109/02699052.2013.830332

Oddy, M., Frances-Moir, J., Fortescue, D., & Chadwick, S. (2012). The prevalence of traumatic brain injury in the homeless community in a UK city. *Brain Injury, 26,* 1058–1064. doi:10.3109/02699052.2012.667595

Oddy, M., & Herbert, C. (2003). Intervention with families following brain injury: Evidence-based practice. *Neuropsychological Rehabilitation, 13,* 259–273. doi:10.1080/09602010244000345

O'Sullivan, M., Glorney, E., Sterr, A., Oddy, M., & Da Silva Ramos, S. (2015). Traumatic brain injury and violent behavior in females: A systematic review. *Aggression and Violent Behavior, 25,* 54–64. doi:10.1016/j.avb.2015.07.006

Ownsworth, T. L., McFarland, K., & Young, R. M. (2000). Self-awareness and psychosocial functioning following acquired brain injury: An evaluation of a group support programme. *Neuropsychological Rehabilitation, 10,* 465–484. doi:10.1080/09602010050143559

Pace, G. M., Schlund, M. W., Hazard-Haupt, T., Christensen, J. R., Lashno, M., McIver, J., … Morgan, K. A. (1999). Characteristics and outcomes of a home and community-based neurorehabilitation programme. *Brain Injury, 13,* 535–546. doi:10.1080/026990599121430

Parker, J. (2006). *Good practice in brain injury case management.* London, UK: Jessica Kingsley.

Perlesz, A., Kinsella, G., & Crowe, S. (1999). Impact of traumatic brain injury on the family: A critical review. *Rehabilitation Psychology, 44,* 6–35. doi:10.1037/0090-5550.44.1.6

Pessar, L. F., Coad, M. L., Linn, R. T., & Willer, B. S. (1993). The effects of parental traumatic brain injury on the behaviour of parents and children. *Brain Injury, 7,* 231–240. doi:10.3109/02699059309029675

Petersen, H., & Sanders, S. (2015). Caregiving and traumatic brain injury: Coping with grief and loss. *Health and Social Work, 40,* 325–328. doi:10.1093/hsw/hlv063

Ponsford, J., Schönberger, M., & Rajaratnam, S. M. W. (2015). A model of fatigue following traumatic brain injury. *Journal of Head Trauma Rehabilitation, 30,* 277–282. doi:10.1097/htr.0000000000000049

Powell, T. (1997). *Head injury: A practical guide.* London, UK: Speechmark.

Powell, T., Ekin-Wood, A., & Collin, C. (2007). Post-traumatic growth after head injury: A long-term follow-up. *Brain Injury, 21,* 31–38. doi:10.1080/02699050601106245

Prigatano, G. P. (1991). The relationship of frontal lobe damage to diminished awareness: Studies in rehabilitation. In H. S. Levin, H. M. Eisenberg, & A. L. Benton (Eds.), *Frontal lobe function and dysfunction,* (pp. 381–397). New York, NY: Oxford University Press.

Prigatano, G. P. (2005). Disturbances of self-awareness and rehabilitation of patients with traumatic brain injury: A 20-year perspective. *The Journal of Head Trauma Rehabilitation, 20,* 19–29. doi:10.1097/00001199-200501000-00004

Prigatano, G. P. (2008). *Anosognosia and the process and outcome of neurorehabilitation: Cognitive neurorehabilitation. Evidence and application,* (2nd ed.). New York, NY: Cambridge University Press.

Radford, K., Phillips, J., Drummond, A., Sach, T., Walker, M., Tyerman, A., … Jones, T. (2013). Return to work after traumatic brain injury: Cohort comparison and economic evaluation. *Brain Injury, 27,* 507–520. doi:10.3109/02699052.2013.766929

Rohling, M. L., Faust, M. E., Beverly, B., & Demakis, G. (2009). Effectiveness of cognitive rehabilitation following acquired brain injury: A meta-analytic re-examination of Cicerone et al.'s (2000, 2005) systematic reviews. *Neuropsychology, 23,* 20–39. doi:10.1037/a0013659

Rowlands, A. (2000). Understanding social support and friendship: Implications for intervention after acquired brain injury. *Brain Impairment, 1,* 151–164. doi:10.1375/brim.1.2.151

Rowlands, A. (2001). Ability or disability? Strengths-based practice in the area of traumatic brain injury. *Families in Society, 82*, 273–286. doi:10.1606/1044-3894.201

Sander, A. M., Caroselli, J. S., High, W. M., Becker, C., Neese, L., & Scheibel, R. (2002). Relationship of family functioning to progress in a post-acute rehabilitation programme following traumatic brain injury. *Brain Injury, 16*, 649–657. doi:10.1080/02699050210128889

Schneider, V. (2010). Submission to the productivity commission's inquiry into disability care and support. *Brain Injury Australia.* Retrieved from http://www.pc.gov.au/inquiries/completed/disability-support/report

Schönberger, M., Humle, F., & Teasdale, T. W. (2006). The development of the therapeutic working alliance, patients' awareness and their compliance during the process of brain injury rehabilitation. *Brain Injury, 20*, 445–454. doi:10.1080/02699050600664772

Scott, D. (2009). Think child, think family: How adult specialist services can support children at risk of abuse and neglect. *Family Matters, 81*, 37–42.

Segal, D. (2010). Exploring the importance of identity following acquired brain injury: A review of the literature. *International Journal of Child, Youth and Family Studies, 1*(3–4), 293–314.

Shiroma, E. J., Ferguson, P. L., & Pickelsimer, E. E. (2012). Prevalence of traumatic brain injury in an offender population: A meta-analysis. *Journal of Head Trauma Rehabilitation, 27*, E1–E10. doi:10.1097/htr.0b013e3182571c14

Shorland, J., & Douglas, J. M. (2010). Understanding the role of communication in maintaining and forming friendships following traumatic brain injury. *Brain Injury, 24*, 569–580. doi:10.3109/02699051003610441

Simpson, G. K., & Baguley, I. J. (2012). Prevalence, correlates, mechanisms, and treatment of sexual health problems after traumatic brain injury: A scoping review. *Critical Reviews in Physical and Rehabilitation Medicine, 24*, 1–34. doi:10.1615/critrevphysrehabilmed.v24.i1-2.10

Simpson, G. K., Simons, M., & McFadyen, M. (2002). The challenges of a hidden disability: Social work practice in the field of traumatic brain injury. *Australian Social Work, 55*, 24–37. doi:10.1080/03124070208411669

Simpson, G. K., & Tate, R. L. (2007). Suicidality in people surviving a traumatic brain injury: Prevalence, risk factors and implications for clinical management. *Brain Injury, 21*, 1335–1351. doi:10.1080/02699050701785542

Skippon, R. (2013). Supporting families and parenting after parental brain injury. In G. Newby, R. Coetzer, A. Daisley, & S. Weatherhead (Eds.), *Practical neuropsychological rehabilitation in acquired brain injury: A guide for working clinicians,* (pp. 295–322). London, UK: Karnac.

Stuss, D. T., Murphy, K. J., Binns, M. A., & Alexander, M. P. (2003). Staying on the job: The frontal lobes control individual performance variability. *Brain, 126*, 2363–2380. doi:10.1093/brain/awg237

Summerfield, P. (2011). *Serious case review executive summary in respect of Child H.* North Tyneside, UK: North Tyneside Local Safeguarding Children Board.

Tam, S., McKay, A., Sloan, S., & Ponsford, J. (2015). The experience of challenging behaviours following severe TBI: A family perspective. *Brain Injury, 29*, 813–821. doi:10.3109/02699052.2015.1005134

Teasell, R., Bayona, N., Marshall, S., Cullen, N., Bayley, M., Chundamala, J., … Tu, L. (2007). A systematic review of the rehabilitation of moderate to severe acquired brain injuries. *Brain Injury, 21*, 107–112. doi:10.1080/02699050701201524

Temkin, N. R., Corrigan, J. D., Dikmen, S. S., & Machamer, J. (2009). Social functioning after traumatic brain injury. *The Journal of Head Trauma Rehabilitation, 24*, 460–467. doi:10.1097/htr.0b013e3181c13413

Tiar, A. M. V., & Dumas, J. E. (2015). Impact of parental acquired brain injury on children: Review of the literature and conceptual model. *Brain Injury, 29*, 1005–1017. doi:10.3109/02699052.2014.976272

Trahan, E., Pepin, M., & Hopps, S. (2006). Impaired awareness of deficits and treatment adherence among people with traumatic brain injury or spinal cord injury. *Journal of Head Trauma Rehabilitation, 21*, 226–235. doi:10.1097/00001199-200605000-00003

Turner-Stokes, L. (2008). Evidence for the effectiveness of multi-disciplinary rehabilitation following acquired brain injury: A synthesis of two systematic approaches. *Journal of Rehabilitation Medicine, 40*, 691–701. doi:10.2340/16501977-0265

Turner-Stokes, L., Disler, P. B., Nair, A., & Wade, D. T. (2005). Multi-disciplinary rehabilitation for acquired brain injury in adults of working age. *Cochrane Database of Systematic Reviews*. Retrieved from http://www.cochrane.org/CD004170/INJ_rehabilitation-adults-working-age-who-have-brain-injury

Uysal, S., Hibbard, M. R., Robillard, D., Pappadopulos, E., & Jaffe, M. (1998). The effect of parental traumatic brain injury on parenting and child behavior. *Journal of Head Trauma Rehabilitation, 13*, 57–71. doi:10.1097/00001199-199812000-00007

Webb, D. (1998). A "revenge" on modern times: Notes on traumatic brain injury. *Sociology, 32*, 541–555. doi:10.1017/s003803859800008x

Webster, G., & Daisley, A. (2007). Including children in family-focused acquired brain injury rehabilitation: A national survey of rehabilitation staff practice. *Clinical Rehabilitation, 21*, 1097–1108. doi:10.1177/0269215507079833

Willer, B., & Corrigan, J. D. (1994). Whatever it takes: A model for community-based services. *Brain Injury, 8*, 647–659. doi:10.3109/02699059409151017

Winstanley, J., Simpson, G., Tate, R., & Myles, B. (2006). Early indicators and contributors to psychological distress in relatives during rehabilitation following severe traumatic brain injury: Findings from the brain injury outcomes study. *Journal of Head Trauma Rehabilitation, 21*, 453–466. doi:10.1097/00001199-200611000-00001

Wood, R. L., McCrea, J. D., Wood, L. M., & Merriman, R. N. (1999). Clinical and cost effectiveness of post-acute neurobehavioural rehabilitation. *Brain Injury, 13*, 69–88. doi:10.1080/026990599121746

Wood, R. L., & Yurdakul, L. K. (1997). Change in relationship status following traumatic brain injury. *Brain Injury, 11*, 491–501. doi:10.1080/bij.11.7.491.501

Worthington, A. D., Matthews, S., Melia, Y., & Oddy, M. (2006). Cost-benefits associated with social outcome from neurobehavioural rehabilitation. *Brain Injury, 20*, 947–957. doi:10.1080/02699050600888314

Mindful Connections: The Role of a Peer Support Group on the Psychosocial Adjustment for Adults Recovering From Brain Injury

Melissa Cutler, Michelle L. A. Nelson, Maya Nikoloski, and Kerry Kuluski

ABSTRACT

How does participating in a peer support group impact an adult's psychosocial adjustment following brain injury? This question was investigated using a qualitative approach, interviewing patients recruited from an ambulatory care program. Data analysis guided by Bury's sociological framework, biographical disruption and biographical repair, revealed participants' pregroup disrupted sense of self, including subthemes related to intrinsic losses and uncertainty. Enhanced psychosocial adjustment including subthemes described participants' reorientation through shared experience. Finally, a postgroup adapted sense of self including subthemes was characterized by heightened purpose, self-awareness, and acceptance. Findings lend weight to using tailored peer interventions to optimize psychosocial adjustment for this population.

The unique challenges faced by adult survivors recovering from a neurological event, who are of prime working age (18–55 years), has gained increasing attention in research and clinical settings (Keppel & Crowe, 2000; Kruger et al., 2010; Kuluski, Dow, Locock, Lyons, & Lasserson, 2014; Lawrence, 2010; Nalder, Fleming, Cornwell, Shields, & Foster, 2013; Oehring & Oakley, 1994). Neurological rehabilitation interventions are noted for their priority on medical and functional aspects of recovery and less often on psychosocial concerns (Kruger et al., 2010; Röding, Lindstrom, Malms, & Öhman, 2003). Moreover, interventions are also criticized for their predominant focus on an older adult population. Whereas physical challenges might be similar to those of an older cohort, younger adult survivors perceive that they face issues related to their developmental stages that can vary across domains such as career, education, relationships, and caregiving responsibilities (Daniel, Wolfe, Busch, & McKevitt, 2009; Kuluski et al., 2014; Low, Kersen, Ashburn, George, & McLellan, 2003; Morris, 2011; Röding et al., 2003). Survivors often feel frustrated and invisible in rehabilitation programs and after discharge, and lack adequate social support resources and self-confidence to face their premorbid lifestyles, relationships, and communities (Nalder et al., 2013; Röding et al., 2003). Consequently, this group of adults who have had a neurological event see themselves as belonging to a distinct patient group (Lawrence, 2010; Morris, 2011).

Over the course of rehabilitation, survivors of unexpected neurological events express psychosocial needs and "invisible" or hidden changes postevent (Kruger et al., 2010; Lawrence, 2010; Low et al., 2003; Morris, 2011). Consistent with studies on persons of primary work-related age, this group of survivors is typically immersed in and prioritizing vocational and income pursuits, likely caring for dependents (young children or elderly), and actively establishing social, intimate, and sexual relationships. There is a perceived loss of control over one's life as well as an expressed need to reestablish self-identity. Thus, when an adult experiences a sudden neurological event at an unforeseen time in his or her life, the major lifestyle implications and psychosocial impact are perceived to be considerably different than those experienced by an older cohort (Banks & Pearson, 2004; Gill, Sander, Robins, Mazzei, & Struchen, 2011; Kuluski et al., 2014; Medin, Barajas, & Ekberg, 2006; Nalder et al., 2013; Teasell, McRae, & Finestone, 2000).

The sociological concept of *biographical disruption* has been widely used to explain the relationship between the sudden onset of illness and its psycho-social impact on one's expected life trajectory (Bury, 1982; Hubbard & Forbat, 2011; Kuluski et al., 2014; McCarthy & Bauer, 2015; Morris, 2011). Bury's (1982) framework emerged from participant interviews conducted with persons aged 25 to 54 years old who were diagnosed with rheumatoid arthritis. Participants' faced a premature onset of chronic illness, which Bury contended resulted in a "disruptive experience" or "critical situation" characterized by a period of significant uncertainty about one's projected disability, quality of life, and social relationships. Further, it is the unexpected timing of the diagnosis in relation to one's expected life course that causes the disablement or disrupts one's sense of self and outlook regarding expected life circumstances.

Although Bury's (1982) framework developed within the chronic illness population, 'biographical disruption' has been applied successfully to explain how persons experience unexpected onset of disease including stroke (Kuluski et al., 2014), motor neuron disease (Locock, Ziebland, & Dumelow, 2009), and cancer (Hubbard & Forbat, 2011). For instance, Kuluski et al. (2014) found that all participants recovering from stroke experienced an "altered sense of self" characterized primarily by the unexpected and major interruptions to normative life expectations regarding self-identity, family life, work, and social roles.

In addition to the disruption caused by the unexpected or premature onset of disease, Bury's framework might also explain how individuals living with other forms of acquired neurological disability such as multiple sclerosis or traumatic brain injury, where the onset falls within normative working age range, also leads to substantial and multifaceted life changes. In a recent literature review on the transition process from hospital to home for persons with acquired brain injury, findings revealed that patients and caregivers lacked tailored emotional and instrumental supports to effectively mitigate the psychosocial discord experienced during this stage of recovery (Turner, Fleming, Ownsworth, & Cornwell, 2008). Further, the authors contended that future transition-specific research should focus on the development of a comprehensive theoretical framework, and in doing so, provide a foundation on which tailored interventions can be designed.

Bury's (1982) work also considered how individuals responded to their disruptive experience and the factors that contributed to personal and community adaptation and reconstruction of self. He contended that mobilizing social support resources could play a significant role in foster adjustment to an "altered situation" and restore a sense of "normality," a process called *biographical repair.* Bury (1982) concluded, "The presence or absence of a supportive social network may make a significant difference in the course of disablement" (p. 175). These sociological concepts lend critical insight into the psychological journey and hardship that often befalls survivors when faced with events that alter their expected life trajectories. Furthermore, Bury's constructs provide a theoretical foundation to explain how social support interventions, and including peer-based services, promote psychosocial adjustment and adaption to a survivor's unexpected life circumstance (Charmaz, 1995; Faircloth, Boylstein, Rittman, Young, & Gubrium, 2004; Kuluski et al., 2014; Lawrence, 2010).

A growing body of clinical and research studies have demonstrated positive outcomes of peer support initiatives on various psychosocial constructs: increased awareness and adaptation to disability, self-confidence, coping, self-efficacy, and self-management of health behavior (Hancock, 2009; Lundqvist, Linnros, Orlenius, & Samuelsson, 2010; Struchen et al., 2011; Webel, Okonsky, Trompeta, & Holzemer, 2010). Peer groups provide safe and familiar environments whereby postevent challenges and accomplishments can be more readily revealed with greater value among peers. Despite an often broad age range among group members who might present with potentially differing developmental life circumstances, a peer support network fulfills an important emotional and social need following unexpected neurological events (Lawrence, 2010; Morris, 2011; Oehring & Oakley, 1994).

After leaving the hospital and transitioning to home, brain injury survivors face the difficult reality of coping with multiple life circumstances. Current research contends that during this stage of recovery, many feel ill equipped to cope with this adjustment (Morris, 2011; Nalder et al., 2013) and perceive it is an "exciting yet difficult period" necessitating tailored, postdischarge supports (Turner et al., 2008). There is limited understanding of how participating in a peer support group tailored for this transition period and designed for various acquired neurodisabilities might mitigate psychosocial discord. This study applied the theoretical frameworks of biographical disruption and biographical repair to explore from the brain injury survivor's perspective the role of a peer support group on their own psychosocial adjustment during the outpatient, community-based stage of their recovery.

Methods

Setting and participants

The Ambulatory Care Program is located at the Bridgepoint site of Sinai Health System, a Toronto, Canada-based rehabilitation and complex care hospital. The program provides outpatient rehabilitation services for adult patients (18 years and older) who present with complex neurological rehabilitation needs that can be treated within a short-term intensive program. The neuro peer support group is offered as an adjunct to individual social work services offered by the Ambulatory Care Program. Group referrals are made by the inpatient or outpatient interdisciplinary team members. The program's social worker, who is also the group facilitator, meets individually with each potential group member prior to the start date to explore his or her interests, expectations, and appropriateness for the group intervention. In this study, all participants were either concurrently participating in rehabilitation therapy services in the Ambulatory Care Program or were within 6 months of their discharge date from this program.

Inclusion criteria for the study included participants could provide informed consent, were English speaking, could articulate responses to open-ended questions with guidance or prompts provided by a trained interviewer, could withstand a one-on-one interview with a researcher for a minimum of 45 min, had previously participated, and were not currently active in the peer support group.

Procedure

Ethics and recruitment

The study received approval from the Joint Bridgepoint–West Park–Toronto Central Community Care Access Centre Research Ethics Board. Participants were recruited from the Ambulatory Care Program at Sinai Health System–Bridgepoint Site from January 2012 to December 2013.

Recruitment took place at the midterm point of each peer support group; the Ambulatory Care clinical manager (an individual not directly involved in patient care) approached potential participants to provide introductory details of the research study using a preapproved script. If interested, individuals provided their contact information. Interested parties were then contacted by phone by the research interviewer (the third author), who provided further explanation of the study and, with verbal consent, arranged an interview time at a private designated room in the hospital. Prior to commencing the interview, written consent was obtained and any questions or concerns about participation were answered.

Recruitment was drawn from four separate peer support groups or from a total of 30 individuals who attended the group. Each group consisted of 7 to 8 individuals and on average, only half of them expressed interest in participating in the research study. Therefore, the sample was compiled across several groups with the goal of yielding a large enough number to reach saturation and achieve a sample representative of the various types of group members. The sample size was ultimately established once confirmation of theoretical saturation was achieved.

Every group member was given equal opportunity to participate in the study and as mentioned, only those who were interested in the study provided their contact information. Of the total number who agreed to participate, all but one completed the study (one individual did not conduct an interview and withdrew from the study due to personal reasons).

Group overview

Each group consisted of a maximum of 10 patients and was held over eight biweekly sessions, or approximately 16 weeks. Each session was 90 min in duration and took place in a meeting room located within the Ambulatory Care Program setting.

All sessions were facilitated by the Ambulatory Care social worker and every session focused on a particular topic related to living with a brain injury. Sessions began with a brief "check-in" period (i.e., approximately 15 min) where members could share recent problems or accomplishments that occurred in between sessions. Next, a brief review of the prior session's topic was done (i.e., approximately 15 min) and finally, members would reach consensus on the current session agenda.

The initial session was meant to be introductory and began by the facilitator welcoming members and providing an overview of the group format and overarching theme. The facilitator normalized any anxious or nervous feelings about joining a group and reinforced that members could share within their comfort levels. Then the facilitator guided members in generating a list of group norms or "ground rules," and finally they participated in a group exercise to get to know one another. Each member was asked to share his or her story, including aspects of his or her medical event, what each expected from participating in the group, and highlighting something "special" about him or her. This acted as an icebreaker for members, as well as an opportunity for the facilitator to detect any overt interpersonal, behavioral, or communication challenges within the group.

A predetermined list of discussion topics was presented during the first session allowing members to provide input and negotiate the order in which topics were discussed based on priority and interest. Although the list of topics was consistent across groups, natural variation in discussion occurred as a result of participant input and group dynamics. The facilitator also allowed for flexibility in the discussion so that at any time, participants could raise pertinent issues and seek assistance from group members.

Discussion topics were largely related to psychosocial adjustment and included coping with difficult emotions, self-image and self-esteem, relationships and sexuality, stress management, anger management, productivity and activity planning, and returning to vocational and avocational settings. When requested by the group, guest speakers were arranged, including the Ambulatory Care registered nurse and occupational therapist, who presented on nutrition and energy conservation, respectively.

Various strategies were employed throughout the program to compensate for members' cognitive, communication, and behavioral challenges. For example, to address difficulties in memory and new learning, all members were given a folder that contained session handouts and educational material, flyers for community resources and local events, and a schedule of session dates and times. Handouts consisted of summary notes from group exercises and key messages scribed by the facilitator on flip chart paper so members did not have to write during the session. The summary notes were typed in larger font and with extra spaces in between lines to assist with visual and language-based barriers. For certain topics, members were given worksheets as an option to further their understanding of the topic and if written input was required, they were encouraged to seek help from loved ones. Additionally, at the start of each session, the facilitator reviewed the prior session's topic to reinforce key ideas and to elicit any further comments or concerns before proceeding with a new topic. Finally, to assist with recall of session dates, the facilitator telephoned members the week of the session to remind them of and confirm their attendance and to ensure they had prearranged assisted transportation services.

Learning activities were delivered using multiple modalities to address attention and concentration challenges and to preempt cognitive fatigue. For example, visual aids such as a flip chart were placed in front of the group and used to write down members' key points. A whiteboard indicating the session's agenda served as a visual reminder and tool for redirection if needed. Group discussion was the basis for learning activities and included topic-focused group exercises, brainstorming, and didactic presentation of material by the facilitator or guest speaker. Further, the average group size was 7 members, which allowed for diverse perspectives and rich discussion, yet also allowed for greater control over the flow and pace of group discussion. For instance, the facilitator encouraged one member to speak and finish at a time and frequently paused during discussion to summarize content and repeat key messages. A smaller group size also made it easier for the facilitator to gently redirect members who were tangential or had reduced social pragmatics. Finally, although there was no formal break time embedded in the session agenda, the facilitator frequently checked in with members to gauge interest and fatigue level.

Data collection

Qualitative methods are predicated on using an 'open-ended strategy' for obtaining data as a means to allow participants to freely elaborate on their experiences and for researchers to capture the unique verbal account by each participant to get at the essence of his or her lived experience (Elliot & Timulak, 2005). Data were collected from semistructured, in-depth, one-on-one interviews conducted by the third author with prior training in qualitative interviewing methods; she was not directly involved in any of the groups.

The interviewer followed an interview guide developed by the research team, based on an extensive literature review made up of questions to bring about full exploration of the research question: How does participating in a peer support group impact a young adult's psychosocial adjustment following a neurological event? The interviewer began by asking open-ended exploratory questions designed to enhance participant engagement and elicit background information; for example, "Tell me a bit about your injury," "Describe your experience after your injury," and "What supports did you have outside of the hospital?" As the interview progressed, overarching questions were asked: "Tell me about your experience in the group," "Tell me about your experience with other participants in the group," and "What supports did you experience outside of the group?" At the conclusion of each interview, participants were encouraged to add additional comments and were thanked for their participation.

Interviews were conducted between 1 and 6 months after the group was completed. The 6-month period allowed for participants to integrate the information and skills learned from the group, yet within a period of time to ensure retention and richness of their experience.

Participants' electronic and paper-based medical records were reviewed to extract common baseline characteristics of the study's participants, including participant age, gender, marital status, admitting diagnosis, comorbidities, and duration between date of onset and start of group. Participant interviews were audio-recorded and transcribed verbatim into an electronic format and participants were assigned a random number that served as the participant identifier. Participant names and comments containing potentially identifiable participant information were removed from the transcripts and were excluded in the data collection record.

Data analysis

A descriptive-interpretive methodological approach (Elliot & Timulak, 2005) guided the analysis process comprising the following steps:
1. Transcripts were read while listening to the audio record to capture errors and intonations (pauses, tones).
2. Transcripts were then read multiple times by a designated research assistant who generated analytic memos, notes of significant phrases, statements, and verbatim participant quotations. This 'preanalysis' enhanced the assistant's familiarity with the data, generating initial impressions, including the overall meaning and usefulness of the information collected. The research assistant also assessed whether theoretical saturation had been met or if additional interviews were required.

A list of significant statements (nonrepetitive, not overlapping) from each transcript was developed and then grouped into larger units (themes). A coding framework was developed containing both expected themes (e.g., those that relate to the conceptual framework, such as psychosocial adjustment and being a young survivor) and emergent themes (those that are not expected from the outset). Because the expected themes from the conceptual framework were based on theoretical and empirical research, the analysis is considered directed content analysis and enabled the researchers to test the robustness of this framework (Kuluski et al., 2014).

The first and fourth authors independently reviewed the coding framework and then met with the research assistant to collectively discuss the findings and reach consensus on differing points of view. Researchers disclosed their pre-research ideas and preconceptions of the phenomenon as a means of minimizing bias and to ensure that themes emerged as part of the interpretive design. The themes were entered into a data software program (NVivo 9) and organized into categories (nodes) for the purpose of extracting the common elements of the experience. This software program enhanced the researchers' ease of accessing the data, auditing, and tracking the emerging results with the original data set throughout the analysis process. Once all data were coded, text from all interviews that fell under each category was gathered and read. The first author and third author independently read through the categories and grouped them into broader themes using axial coding (a process of relating and grouping codes).

Based on the timing of the groups and subsequent interview dates, transcripts from 11 participants were initially analyzed. It was determined that theoretical saturation was achieved; however, given that data from the five remaining interviews were not yet included in the analysis, the researchers decided to use the data to confirm saturation was reached and this was the case with minor variation in themes.

A summary was written for each theme, aiming to capture all experiences, including key themes by volume of response. Finally, a detailed description of the phenomenon was created, based on the themes and participant quotations, as well as containing the shared elements of the participants' experiences. The application to existing literature and Bury's (1982) theoretical framework was discussed. Additional questions and future research directions were identified.

Results

Participants' demographic characteristics are detailed in Table 1. The accounting of such personal health information enabled researchers to examine pertinent features of the survivor profile not captured during the interview. As indicated in Table 1, 7 men and 9 women were interviewed. The age range was 23 to 54 years at the time of the interview and the average age of the participants was 41.4 years old. All participants had a primary neurological diagnosis and 9 out of 16 participants (over 50%) presented with comorbidities. The majority of participants were within 1 year of their event and some were up to 3 years postevent.

The sample's broad age range suggests that participants were possibly dealing with developmentally specific life circumstances that could be tied to differing psychosocial challenges. Despite this external factor, core themes related to biographical disruption and biographical repair were extrapolated based on shared group experiences.

Through interpretation of participants' interview responses, the meaning of participating in a peer support group on the psychosocial adjustment for brain injury survivors emerged. Three principal themes, each with subthemes, were identified and are summarized in Table 2. The first theme, disrupted sense of self, included three subthemes: loss of identity, living with uncertainty, and social isolation. The second theme, enhanced psychosocial adjustment, revealed seven subthemes, including motivating effect, validation and normalization of experiences, social connection and reintegration, sense of routine and structure, socially accepted sharing, information sharing and skills building, and stepping stone toward normalcy. Finally, an adapted sense of self emerged as a third broad theme consisting of three subthemes: reality check, restored purpose, and enhanced self-acceptance.

Disrupted sense of self

When asked what their experience was like before joining the group, most participants expressed feeling "lost" postevent, characterized by difficulties adjusting to a significant disruption and disorientation to their normal daily living. For example, participants shared their inability to resume premorbid social roles including working, driving, socializing, living independently, and juggling family and life responsibilities. In addition to adjusting to functional limitations, all participants struggled with the psychological cost of role loss and diminished

Table 1. Summary of participant characteristics.

Participant no.	Age at onset	Gender	Marital status	Admitting diagnosis	Comorbidities	Date of onset[a] (from start of group)
P1	42	M	Single	Multifocal motor neuropathy	Depression	4
P2	50	F	Divorced	Stroke	N/A	2
P3	45	M	Common law	Brain tumor	N/A	4
P4	53	F	Common law	Brain tumor	Diabetes mellitus; hypertension; hyperthyroid	1
P5	51	M	Married	Stroke	New onset diabetes mellitus; hypertension; hyperlipidemia	1
P6	50	M	Married	TBI	Depression	3
P7	54	F	Divorced	TBI	N/A	3
P8	27	M	Single	Epilepsy, lobectomy	Depression	1
P9	30	F	Married	Multiple sclerosis flare-up	N/A	1
P10	23	M	Single	Stroke	Anxiety	1
P11	30	F	Single	Multiple sclerosis flare-up	N/A	1
P12	45	F	Single	Stroke		1
P13	43	F	Single	1. Pulmonary embolism, cardiac arrest, seizures; 2. Secondary progressive multiple sclerosis	Depression	3
P14	46	F	Married	Multiple sclerosis	Depression and anxiety	1
P15	47	M	Divorced	TBI	Diabetes mellitus	2
P16	27	F	Common law	Stroke		2

Note: TBI = traumatic brain injury.
[a]1 = 0–6 months; 2 = 6–12 months, 3 = 1–2 years, 4 = > 2 years.

Table 2. Summary of core themes, subthemes, and thematic descriptions.

Core theme	Subthemes
Disrupted sense of self	Loss of identity
	The inability to resume social roles, increased dependency on loved ones, magnifying diminished self-sufficiency and inadequacy
	Living with uncertainty
	Uncertain futures, amplified feelings of self-doubt and low self-esteem
	Social isolation
	Participants could no longer relate to existing supports; social outlets were inaccessible and fear of overburdening supports emerged
Enhanced psychosocial adjustment	Motivating effect
	Participants thrived off each other's successes, building confidence to face their own challenges
	Validation and normalization of experiences
	Participants gained emotional support from shared understanding and relating to others facing similar experiences
	Social connection and reintegration
	The group was a relevant and meaningful social activity replacing lost social opportunities and mitigating some withdrawal
	Sense of routine and structure
	Participants reestablished a sense of structure by committing continuously to a set time and place
	Socially accepted sharing
	The group was a "safe," nonjudgmental forum in which to speak freely and articulate experiences
	Information sharing and skills building
	Participants valued shared knowledge building, coping, and life skills
	Stepping stone toward normalcy
	The group provided a first step toward transitioning to the "outside world"
Adapted sense of self	Reality check
	Participants expanded self-perspective by comparing their situation with peers, yielding gratitude and humility
	Restored purpose
	Participants were empowered by sharing stories, providing purpose and social value
	Enhanced self-acceptance
	The group experience led to enhanced adaptation and self-determination despite current circumstances and uncertain futures

social involvement. Participants spoke of "invisible" changes, namely, cognitive, emotional, psychological, and social changes that led to feelings of diminished social value, sense of purpose, and uncertainty over their recovery potential and reintegrating into larger society. Moreover, the intrinsic 'loss' felt by participants was difficult to articulate to family and friends and amplified feelings of loneliness, self-doubt, and disconnect from emotional and social supports. For many, these effects were unrealized or not openly expressed until they reached the peer group. Subthemes and supporting quotations are explored further here.

Loss of identity

As stated earlier, when one experiences a sudden and unexpected neurological event at a time in his or her life that could be considered "prime," it can have major lifestyle and psychological implications. For instance, all participants held and identified with multiple social roles. All were actively pursuing professional careers or academic degrees or building existing ones. Some were recently married, dating, involved in significant relationships, and parents to young children or caring for elders. In the following text, a 30-year-old woman recently diagnosed with multiple sclerosis and in the hospital for a related flare-up described the disruption and significant impact of the event on her chosen lifestyle and social roles. As shown in Table 1, P9 stands for Participant 9, P7 for Participant 7, and so on.

> Before I got sick, I worked in a job that was very stressful, very intense but I always felt like, you know, I was sort of needed in my job. Like I would work crazy hours and push myself too hard but I felt like, you know, my purpose was I'd go to work and get the stuff done and be effective at it, and be a good boss. And then when I got sick and I left my job, I mean that … I was lost. Like where do I go from here? Like I am a newly married person who is planning to have a family soon, and that's off the table right now. My job is off the table right now. You sort of are like what's the point? Like what is my purpose. (P9)

In the transition to home and living in the community, many participants were adjusting to reduced independence to complete their personal care or activities of daily living. Daily tasks once deemed easy and part of their "role" were either abandoned or being completed by a combination of informal or formal supports. Although appreciation for instrumental support was expressed by all participants, it was often marred by conflicting feelings of personal inadequacy and frustration over unforeseen dependency and diminished daily purpose and sense of productivity. Some participants were faced with reversing roles with family members for whom they once were the primary caregivers. As described by a participant on her continued adjustment 1 year after her traumatic neurological event:

> It's not great. Not great because of that. Because you know, my parents are 82 and 86. And this is not the normal course of events. I'm not supposed to be under their care you know. … And psychologically it wasn't good because this is not how life is supposed to happen. (P7)

The realization that participants might be forced to abandon or modify their socially valued and self-identifying roles was viewed as an added psychological blow to their sense of selves. The threat that things were not "normal" anymore and the perceived inability to resume meaningful roles became a harsh reality. The following quotation describes one participant's struggle with self-identity postevent:

> Because in my case, I spent 54 years living as a certain person and now all of a sudden, I now have to function as somebody who is different. And it is very odd. Like there are some things I don't change, you know, we have a certain personality. But I mean there are things by which I identify myself which no longer exist. And I didn't even realize that this is how I presented myself to the world

and this is how I functioned within it because these things were so important and so much a part of who I was. (P7)

Similarly, a 53-year-old woman diagnosed with a brain tumor described the sudden impact on her sense of self.

> Sometimes, you know, you were faced with very hard situations because it's not easy being, you know, all of a sudden illness hits you and you're this way, completely the opposite. (P4)

Living with uncertainty

Participants felt ill equipped to cope with the uncertainty of their recovery potential, not knowing how their current circumstances would impact their future quality of life. As they transitioned from the hospital to living in the community, participants relied on their premorbid self-expectations as a guide for reintegrating into their former lives and relationships. When attempts to resume premorbid activities failed or their performance was significantly different than their expectations, participants' sense of disruption and self-doubt regarding their adjustment amplified. As described by a 46-year-old mother of young children,

> I'd been home for maybe a month or two. And still struggling with the fact that I'm off work and feeling guilty for not being back at work. And still expecting my ability to do all the things that I used to do as a mom to be there. And yet my energy wasn't there yet. And I was really struggling a lot with just coming to terms with my new reality and not even realizing what it was sometimes. (P14)

Participants expressed having to adjust to the reality that future goals and life plans articulated before their events were "put on hold" or were perceived as indefinitely delayed. Living with the uncertainty brought on by a sudden event was illustrated in the case of a participant living with progressive multiple sclerosis.

> You feel like when something comes on like this, like your life just completely turns upside down. And all the things that you've kind of worked for in your life, you're wondering what's going to happen. And your future is uncertain. (P9)

Lacking the certainty of when and how much one could recover perpetuated beliefs of poor self-concept and self-esteem. For some participants, this was reflected in their self-care and outlook. As illustrated by a 45-year-old stroke survivor,

> Because I'm actually quite … usually a very positive person and glass half full. And then I got depressed. I really did. And I mean I was lucky, I never lost my ability to walk. But I lost some vision and I couldn't drive. And I was just tired, fatigued, and I didn't care about anything. And so I began to think … Like I didn't care about clothes, I didn't care about makeup, I didn't care how I looked. I didn't care anything. And so you think at the time that's my new me. I'm never going to care. I'm never going to want to buy clothes. I'm never going to care about makeup. I'm never going to, you know, care about things I used to care about. And so you're in this thing. (P12)

Social isolation

Reduced independence and reliance on others magnified participants' perceptions of their diminished self-sufficiency. Subsequently, changes in social relationships and roles emerged, including difficulties connecting with loved ones whom they now felt were unexpectedly saddled with being their caregivers. Hesitation to reach out on a social level was driven by participants' worry about overburdening existing supports.

> So it wasn't like sitting at home with my husband who's incredibly supportive but you feel bad after a while with talking about like I'm struggling with this or I'm struggling with this. Like you want to make sure that you don't do that so much that you drive people in your life away. (P9)

Participants had difficulty in relating to friends and family who were not experiencing similar lifestyle changes. Daily struggles, concerns, and priorities were different than prior to their event, causing disconnect in participants' relationships and their interactions. A 23-year-old man described the social disconnect in his life before joining the group:

> It's harder to connect to people out in the real world because it's like well, they are so stressed out with exams and I'm dealing with having five grand mal seizures. There's a bit of a disconnect. Whereas people in the peer group kind of have that risk and they know what it's like to live in that fear. (P10)

Finally, for many participants, work, school, and recreational environments were naturally occurring social outlets no longer available or accessible due to finances, motivation, or transportation. Participants were also concerned about how others would perceive them if they partook in these activities. The significant impact of recovering from brain surgery on one's social life is described here by a participant:

> So much of my social scene was around, you know, meeting folks at the bar. And now it's like a complete … It turns it on its head. It means that I need to find new friends or I can't rely on them to call me out to join them because they're uncomfortable with it or maybe I'm not as fun when I'm sober. So that's been a big effect. (P8)

Enhanced psychosocial adjustment

In the participants' journey from a disrupted to an adapted sense of self, the group provided a venue for enhancing participants' psychosocial adjustment. The group offered a socially relevant and consistent meeting place that helped participants to build structure and purpose in their daily routines. It provided a platform for participants to speak freely and to feel understood and validated. The ability to connect with peers at similar developmental stages also had significant emotional and social value. Participants' enhanced psychosocial adjustment emerged through seven subthemes including motivating effect, validation and normalization of experiences, social connection and reintegration, sense of routine and structure, socially accepted sharing, information sharing and skills building, and stepping stone toward normalcy.

Motivating effect

Participants were motivated by listening to other participants' stories of overcoming everyday challenges in their journey to establish a "new normal" since returning to the community. The belief prevailed that if one member could overcome challenges in his or her own personal life, then they, too, could rise to the challenge in their own lives. The act of sharing personal accomplishments and triumphs increased participants' self-confidence and comfort level to face tasks they might not have considered possible prior to joining the group. As shown by the following participant's group experience:

> Because where you're sitting at home and just not feeling well, you feel like you don't have any outlets. But after you came out of the room, it was like wow, look at so and so is doing, and this person does that. You just realize you can take the cap off yourself. You have no limits. So those things really helped. (P11)

Validation and normalization of experiences

Participants drew emotional and psychological support from being in a group with people with perceived similar traits despite the broad developmental age range. The opportunity to receive encouragement, feedback, and shared understanding met untapped needs for the validation and the normalization of participants' experiences. Participants valued being understood on their own terms and related to others going through similar experiences. Although many participants were uncertain initially about what to expect from participating in a peer support group, as the group progressed, there was an eventual ease and drawing to one another through mutual sharing and a fundamental understanding that "you were not alone."

> A sense of companionship that I had lost. Finding people that were like me. Finding people that were worse off than me. Finding people that were able to cope with it better than me. Finding people that weren't able to cope with it better than me. Just finding people that knew. That knowing is a beautiful gift. (P10)

Participants also expressed a collective identity and strength that evolved from their group membership. For instance, having a place to voice their worries and victories and then have it be recognized and acknowledged by their peers fostered a sense of accomplishment and ownership. As shared by a participant:

> I remember somebody saying something good, what they were about. And I would kind of like take that on as proud of my achievement as well because I was in this group. Because I'm part of this family and so when so and so did well, that I some way or another, you know I would carry that positive thing with me as well. (P7)

Social connection and reintegration

The group was viewed as an important social gathering, a replacement for social opportunities that were either lost or inaccessible. By virtue of allowing participation in a group setting, the peer support group simulated a "normal" social gathering despite the clinical, hospital environment. For many participants, it was also the first time they had encountered others who were at similar stages of their recovery.

> It was the first time that I've ever been in a setting like that where I could speak openly and have open conversation with people about similar obstacles. Although they were night and day, we still faced things that were a disruption in our lives that we're going to have to live with forever. (P1)

The need to connect with their own peers, who were experiencing similar medical and developmental challenges, was noted among many participants. The outlet helped to mitigate social isolation and withdrawal commonly shared by participants. The group's social value was expressed by one participant:

> And after surgery, you're not exactly keen on taking the initiative to meet new friends and stuff. So the fact that this sort of added on another useful aspect of recovery without having to put in the extra effort to seek out friends and folks to chat with, people who hadn't heard your stories before, and could relate to them better, that was a great benefit. (P8)

Sense of routine and structure

The group provided a scheduled time and meeting place that allowed participants to plan ahead and have an activity they looked forward to. By attending the group, participants took a step toward reestablishing a sense of routine that helped to build structure and a sense of purpose into their daily lives.

> You know what, it provided kind of a bit of a routine in that I had to be at a certain place at a certain time and do a certain thing. And so when you have that, you feel you're doing something. (P7)

Socially acceptable sharing

Participants described the group setting as a "safe," nonjudgmental place where they spoke candidly about their experiences, and many of them shared similar stores. Participants also used the sessions to collectively problem solve and obtain input on presenting issues. Although many had support networks, the group's feedback offered significant value because it was from peers. The value of speaking freely about her hardship is expressed in the following participant quotation:

> We were allowed to be truthful. Sometimes, you know, you were faced with very hard situations because it's not easy being, you know, all of a sudden illness hits you and you're this way, completely the opposite. So it helps. (P4)

Participants also learned how to verbalize their experiences and start to articulate them to others. Subsequently, this process helped members to build self-confidence and to ease their comfort level when faced with future social and interpersonal situations.

> So I mean if you found something that was particularly inspiring that week or a challenge that you overcame, you could talk about that. And that made you feel good about yourself, too, and realizing that, you know, there are things that are positive. And being able to reflect on that and share that with other people let you feel, I guess, needed in a sense, and inspirational rather than just the sick person or the victim or somebody to feel sorry for kind of thing. (P9)

Information sharing and skills building

Participants valued shared knowledge and resources. Participants gained skills to cope with lifestyle changes, relationships, stress, and emotionality. Participants expressed the benefits of learning coping strategies from their peers but also having an opportunity to gain knowledge and handouts from the facilitator on topics regarding brain injury. Having educational materials and resource brochures provided information they could hold onto and review at a future date or share with their loved ones.

> It's always good to have reinforcement and listen to what other people have to say. Sometimes they have tips and things like that. And so it's always good to meet with other people who have different ideas of how they go about things. (P14)

Stepping stone toward normalcy

Although all participants were living in the community, many were adjusting to the "real world," namely, living outside of the protective and supportive hospital environment. The group was viewed as an important component of reintegrating into premorbid lifestyles and most considered it a first step toward transitioning to the "outside world." The interim support provided by the group brought about a normalization and preparation for life reintegration that was not sufficiently provided by family and loved ones. As summarized by a participant comparing the impact of group support with her existing support network:

> It definitely provided the transition between the inside and the outside world. And as much as I have a lot of support myself, it was still not the kind of support that I was receiving here. And by that I mean that, you know, the support that I have are from regular people who have not gone through an incident which is essentially a life altering one for me and the other people that were there as well. (P7)

When the group ended, many participants commented they felt strongly connected to their group peers and viewed them no longer as fellow "patients," but rather as lifelong friends. Such bonds culminated in an internal support network not otherwise present during their recovery. The restored social value grew out of these bonds and propelled participants' psychosocial adjustment.

I have lifelong friends now that I will always keep in contact with. And I just think that it's a good system of support that people can actually find happiness and settlement with their own injuries. (P10)

Adapted sense of self

An adapted sense of self developed through the shared group experience, organically grown via a network of mutual support and understanding. In contrast with premorbid outlook and self-perspective, at the group's end, participants held a broadened awareness and enhanced acceptance of their current circumstances. Propelled by a sense of purpose and giving back, participants found positive meaning in their current state that fostered their psychosocial adjustment despite an unchanged reality. Three subthemes characterized participants' postgroup adapted sense of self, including reality check, restored purpose, and enhanced self-acceptance.

Reality check

Being part of a peer support group provided an opportunity for participants to view their own situation in relation to their developmental peers, many with similar as well as more challenging issues than their own. Most participants entered the group relying only on their own experience as the main reference point for how to cope with their respective events. By listening to member stories and gaining diverse perspectives, participants experienced a "reality check" or self-reflection that, until joining the group, had been overshadowed by the disruption and disorientation left by their events. The reality check acted as a catalyst for expanded awareness as illustrated by a participant's insight:

> It's like everybody has their own struggles and issues and worries that they're worried about. And so I think it kind of took away from like the "poor me, nobody understands" mindset and made you realize that, you know, you're not the only person in the world that struggles and there are other people who have challenges. (P9)

Through the self-reflective process, participants compared their own situations with that of group members, which yielded both gratitude and humility about their own situation. Participants described feeling conflicted when meeting members with more significant impairments, yet were inspired by their resilience in spite of their circumstances. Comparison of stories, in part, had a positive impact on participants' self-perspective by challenging their own beliefs about their capabilities and sense of self. Participants could also reflect on their own strength in the context of their perceived disrupted life course. Subsequently, by grounding in their personal situation, participants' pregroup lens was broadened and an expanded view and meaning of their own situation emerged. Here a participant acknowledged a shift in her self-perception at the group's end.

I mean in some cases it made count myself lucky. Things could be worse unfortunately when you see, you know, that other people have it worse than you. But it was also amazing to see how other people cope with things that are worse than you. (P14)

Similarly, a 23-year-old stroke survivor also reflected on the unexpected positive impact on his self-awareness when considering others' hardships.

So I needed to meet people that have had if not as bad as me, if not worse. Which meeting the people that had it worse than me made me very humble about my own incident. Which was a very good experience because it made me stop talking about it so much, like my life isn't that tragic compared to some of these people. (P10)

Restored purpose

Participants felt empowered by helping others through sharing their personal stories, successes, and ongoing struggles. At a time in their recovery when diminished role involvement and loss of identity prevailed, participants adopted a "pay it forward" perspective during the group experience. Participants developed an unanticipated compassion and motivation to help others in the group whom they perceived were in worse circumstances. This "helper role," in part, restored a sense of purpose and social value for participants. One participant reflected on his group experience as a means for empowering his own sense of self and in turn, positioning himself to help future survivors.

And I know it's horrible to take that from them but they're making my life better. Which I hope I can demonstrate to them some day that they've helped somebody. And I hope to help somebody from my experience as well. Like pay it forward, as it were. (P10)

The ability to make valuable contributions within a socially relevant setting was intrinsically rewarding and perhaps acted as a protective factor against further psychosocial stress. The connections between value-added sharing, renewed self-worth, and an adapted sense of self are illustrated in the following quotation:

So being in a group where you feel like you can add value and have a bit of an influence on people and feel like okay, maybe there is a purpose, even if it's a little one, just for now it gives you something to sort of hold onto ... which is at that point everything. Like have a meaning and having a purpose I think prevents you from becoming severely depressed. (P9)

Enhanced self-acceptance

As participants moved toward a more insightful and adaptive way of living, feelings of self-pity, disruption, and stagnation decreased while enhanced adaptation and self-determination to push despite current circumstances emerged. As explained by a 47-year-old participant recovering from a motor vehicle collision,

I mean so if these people could accept the reality and they cope with it, well, of course I said I can do it myself. So well, this is strong personalities surround me so I made myself stronger. (P15)

Similarly, another participant shared feelings of restored hope and motivation attributed to emerging self-acceptance despite her diagnosis and uncertain future.

It gives me that hope that, wow, you know, there's no reason to be afraid of this disease and, you know, people do cope with things worse than what I've experienced. (P14)

Despite an unchanged reality and uncertainty around their recovery and future quality of life, self-acceptance counteracted self-perceptions of inadequacy and dependency. At the group's end, participants felt internally better equipped and self-determined to move forward in their lives. As shared by a participant's reflections at the group's end,

So I learned two things. It's either you sit down and whine about it or you pick yourself up and you move on. So basically the group, it teaches me that what I learn is that you've got to move on. Right? So that's the main problem with me—accepting that life is not going to be like it is before. Right? And then the second thing, to make that adjustment. (P3)

Participants' enhanced self-acceptance meant they could move forward and work toward a more realistic way of living and coming to terms with their situation. For many participants, this involved reconstructing their view of themselves, namely, accepting and incorporating the event's impact but not exclusively being defined by it. As described by a stroke survivor:

And it gives me an acceptance because like these things happened to me but they don't define who I am. I am who I am. And they have changed who I am but they don't define who I am. Which is nice. Like it's really given me kind of a wake-up call. (P10)

Discussion

This study demonstrated that participating in a peer support group designed for adult brain injury survivors during the outpatient rehabilitation phase fostered participants' psychosocial adjustment. Participants presented themselves to the group with a disrupted sense of self characterized by feelings of diminished self-worth and social value. Features of enhanced psychosocial adjustment surfaced through mutual sharing of similar experiences whereby participants garnered validation and normalization of feelings of loss and uncertainty not fully expressed until joining the group. Finally, an adapted sense of self emerged whereby participants broadened their insight and self-acceptance of their current circumstances despite facing an unchanged reality.

The application of the theoretical frameworks for biographical disruption and biographical repair was relevant in this study. For instance, participants' pregroup disrupted self-perception aligned with Bury's (1982) concept of biographical disruption, whereby the suddenness and unexpected nature of a traumatic event interrupts one's sense of self, self-identity, and life circumstances. Participants' pregroup perspectives were tied to their former social roles and relationships (which had been diminished or lost since their injuries). Subsequently, participants expressed a lack of purpose, intrinsic loss, and social value. These findings expand recent literature demonstrating that survivors at prime working age lack targeted (Morris, 2011) postdischarge services (Turner et al., 2008), experience an "altered sense of self" (Kuluski et al., 2014), and face identity changes (Nalder et al., 2013) on transitioning to the community.

Shared elements revealed by this study highlight the positive association between peer support groups, psychosocial adjustment, and interventions targeted for the brain injury population. Previous research consistently demonstrated that peer support initiatives positively affect psychosocial adjustment following a traumatic health event (Lundqvist et al., 2010; Struchen et al., 2011; Webel et al., 2010), yet also stressed incongruence between identifying survivors' needs and providing age-appropriate and tailored services following brain injury (Lawrence, 2010; Morris, 2011; Turner et al., 2008). This study determined to bridge such gaps and expanded our understanding of this phenomenon.

Participants' postgroup adapted sense of self highlighted elements of biographical repair through a dynamic and shared process of naming and validating feelings, and counteracting self-perceptions of inadequacy and dependence. In line with previous research, the group acted as a venue for sharing experiences related to participants' adjustment and was a pivotal step in their adaptation and changed perspective of their outside world (Charmaz, 1995; Nalder et al., 2013). Participants maintained uncertainty over the future, yet gained purpose, insight, and social acceptance, which fostered participants' self-confidence and self-determination to cope with current circumstances.

Clinical application and future research

This study examined the meaning of a peer support group intervention within a specific and time-limited episode of care during the outpatient community-based stage of recovery. The majority of participants joined the group within the first year of their injuries. Consideration of future research to examine how survivors cope at latter stages of their rehabilitation might inform how peer interventions foster long-term psychosocial adjustment beyond the first year of recovery. Longitudinal research would further reveal information on survivors' psychosocial needs at different rehabilitation transitional points and when to provide peer interventions.

Given the marked psychosocial disruption experienced by participants prior to joining the peer support group, consideration in future research should be given to exploring the impact of providing such groups as part of an inpatient rehabilitation program. As this study targeted high-functioning survivors, its clinical application is only intended for this subset of the brain injury population. Future examination of the psychosocial needs of adult survivors presenting with a continuum of injury impairments might inform how peer groups apply to a wider spectrum of brain injury survivors.

Participants' feedback regarding opportunities for improving the group is noteworthy for developing its future application and benefits. Many participants commented on the stark, clinical setting of the group and desired the sessions to take place in a more "organic," social setting like a nearby coffee shop, local park, or community center. It was felt that if the group was conducted in a location that was detached from the hospital environment, then it might boost the group's natural social value. In terms of the group structure and session format, some participants expressed wanting a "warmup" period at the start of the sessions to improve their comfort level within the group context. Some participants also expected to be given homework tasks to maintain momentum in between sessions. No specific suggestions were made regarding discussion topics; however, many suggested inviting a former group member to a session, as someone who could potentially offer further perspective and inspiration on coping with the recovery process. These recommendations can be used to adapt the current programming in place and might be useful for other providers who are looking to start or refine support groups for this population.

Limitations

There are some limitations to this study. The participants represented a subset of high-functioning neurological survivors and thus did not include survivors with significant impairments (which by design would have excluded such patients from participating in the peer support group). These findings are applicable to those patients who present with similar impairments. This study explored survivors' psychosocial adjustment at specific times in their recovery whereby the findings should be considered within this defined episode of care.

As suggested previously, consideration of future research examining psychosocial adjustment across all transition points during neurological recovery would yield valuable insight into developmental age and rehabilitation stage-specific interventions. Finally, the intent of the research was not to test the effectiveness of the support group, but rather to use the group as a venue to understand how people adjust to psychosocial challenges postevent. As such, participants' adjustment might have also resulted from factors occurring outside of the group experience.

Conclusion

The findings reported here expand current understanding of the psychosocial adjustment process for adult brain injury survivors. They underscore the clinical significance of taking a holistic approach to neurological rehabilitation services that incorporate the psychosocial needs of younger adult patients including when they transition to the community. Peer support groups could bridge a widening gap in current rehabilitation services by offering a forum for mutual psychosocial support, a key component of social, emotional, and community reintegration. Designing tailored interventions that address psychosocial challenges could facilitate long-term adjustment and preempt prolonged psychosocial distress for this set of survivors.

Acknowledgments

The authors would like to thank Sylvia Hoang, Mary McAllister, and Jennifer Spencer for their earlier contributions to this study. We would also like to thank the 16 participants for volunteering their time and sharing their experiences with brain injury.

References

Banks, P., & Pearson, C. (2004). Parallel lives: Younger stroke survivors and their partners coping with crisis. *Sexual and Relationship Therapy, 19*, 413–429. doi:10.1080/14681990412331298009

Bury, M. (1982). Chronic illness as biographical disruption. *Sociology of Health and Illness, 4*, 167–182.

Charmaz, K. (1995). The body, identity, and self: Adapting to impairment. *Sociological Quarterly, 36*, 657–680. doi:10.1111/j.1533-8525.1995.tb00459.x

Daniel, K., Wolfe, C. D. A., Busch, M. A., & McKevitt, C. (2009). What are the social consequences of stroke for working-aged adults? A systemic review. *Stroke, 40*, e431–e440. doi:10.1161/strokeaha.108.534487

Elliot, R., & Timulak, L. (2005). Descriptive and interpretive approaches to qualitative research. In J. Miles & P. Gilbert (Eds.), *A handbook of research methods for clinical and health psychology* (pp. 147–159). New York, NY: Oxford University Press.

Faircloth, C. A., Boylstein, C., Rittman, M., Young, M. E., & Gubrium, J. (2004). Sudden illness and biographical flow in narratives of stroke recovery. *Sociology of Health and Illness, 26*, 242–261. doi:10.1111/j.1467-9566.2004.00388.x

Gill, C. J., Sander, A. M., Robins, N., Mazzei, D. K., & Struchen, M. A. (2011). Exploring experiences of intimacy from the viewpoint of individuals with traumatic brain injury and their partners. *Journal of Head Trauma Rehabilitation, 26*(1), 56–68. doi:10.1097/htr.0b013e3182048ee9

Hancock, E. (2009, May). *Health recovery social networks: Exploring the experiences of participants in stroke recovery peer support groups.* Paper presented at the Association for Non-Profit and Social Economy Research annual conference, Ottawa, ON, Canada.

Hubbard, G., & Forbat, L. (2011). Cancer as biographical disruption: Constructions of living with cancer. *Supportive Care in Cancer, 20*, 2033–2040. doi:10.1007/s00520-011-1311-9

Keppel, C. C., & Crowe, S. F. (2000). Changes to body image and self-esteem following stroke in young adults. *Neuropsychological Rehabilitation, 10*(1), 15–31. doi:10.1080/096020100389273

Kruger, H., Graham, J. R., Kruger, E., Teasell, R., Foley, N., & Salter, K. (2010). *The rehabilitation of younger stroke patients.* London, ON, Canada: Canadian Stroke Network.

Kuluski, K., Dow, C., Locock, L., Lyons, R. F., & Lasserson, D. (2014). Life interrupted and life regained? Coping with stroke at a young age. *International Journal of Qualitative Studies on Health and Well-Being, 9*, 1–12. doi:10.3402/qhw.v9.22252

Lawrence, M. (2010). Young adults' experience of stroke: A qualitative review of the literature. *British Journal of Nursing, 19*, 241–248. doi:10.12968/bjon.2010.19.4.46787

Locock, L., Ziebland, S., & Dumelow, C. (2009). Biographical disruption, abruption and repair in the context of motor neuron disease. *Sociology Health & Illness, 31*, 1043–1058. doi:10.1111/j.1467-9566.2009.01176.x

Low, J. T. S., Kersen, P., Ashburn, A., George, S., & McLellan, D. L. (2003). A study to evaluate the met and unmet needs of members belonging to young stroke groups affiliated with the stroke association. *Disability and Rehabilitation, 25*, 1052–1056. doi:10.1080/0963828031000069753

Lundqvist, A., Linnros, H., Orlenius, H., & Samuelsson, K. (2010). Improved self-awareness and coping strategies for patients with acquired brain injury—A group therapy programme. *Brain Injury, 24*, 823–832. doi:10.3109/02699051003724986

McCarthy, M. J., & Bauer, E. (2015). In sickness and in health: Couples coping with stroke across the life span. *Health and Social Work, 40*(3), e92–e100. doi:10.1093/hsw/hlv043

Medin, J., Barajas, J., & Ekberg, K. (2006). Stroke patients' experiences of return to work. *Disability and Rehabilitation, 28*, 1051–1060. doi:10.1080/09638280500494819

Morris, R. (2011). The psychology of stroke in young adults: The roles of service provision and return to work. *Stroke Research and Treatment, 2011*, 1–10. doi:10.4061/2011/534812

Nalder, E., Fleming, J., Cornwell, P., Shields, C., & Foster, M. (2013). Reflections on life: Experiences of individuals with brain injury during the transition from hospital to home. *Brain Injury, 27*, 1294–1303. doi:10.3109/02699052.2013.823560

Oehring, A. K., & Oakley, J. L. (1994). The young stroke patient: A need for specialized group support systems. *Top Stroke Rehabilitation, 1*(1), 25–40.

Röding, J., Lindstrom, B., Malms, J., & Öhman, A. (2003). Frustrated and invisible: Younger stroke patients' experiences of the rehabilitation process. *Disability and Rehabilitation, 25*, 867–874. doi:10.1080/0963828031000122276

Struchen, M. A., Davis, L. C., Bogaards, J. A., Hudler-Hull, T., Clark, A. N., Mazzei, D. M., … Caroselli, J. S. (2011). Making connections after brain injury: Development and evaluation of a social peer-mentoring program for persons with traumatic brain injury. *Journal of Head Trauma Rehabilitation, 26*(1), 4–19. doi:10.1097/htr.0b013e3182048e98

Teasell, R. W., McRae, M. P., & Finestone, H. M. (2000). Social issues in the rehabilitation of younger stroke patients. *Archives of Physical Medicine and Rehabilitation, 81*, 205–209. doi:10.1016/s0003-9993(00)90142-4

Turner, B. J., Fleming, J. M., Ownsworth, T. L., & Cornwell, P. L. (2008). The transition from hospital to home for individuals with acquired brain injury: A literature review and research recommendations. *Disability and Rehabilitation, 30*, 1153–1176. doi:10.1080/09638280701532854

Webel, A. R., Okonsky, J., Trompeta, J., & Holzemer, W. L. (2010). A systemic review of the effectiveness of peer-based interventions on health-related behaviors in adults. *American Journal of Public Health, 100*, 247–253. doi:10.2105/ajph.2008.149419

Holding Resilience in Trust: Working Systemically With Families Following an Acquired Brain Injury

Franca Butera-Prinzi, Nella Charles, and Karen Story

ABSTRACT
The conceptualization of resilience following acquired brain injury needs to remain sensitive to the complex nature and enduring dimensions of trauma, loss, and stress. It is essential that a systemic and dynamic view be maintained with a focus on the key adaptation tasks that families face: grieving, restructuring, identity redefinition, and growing through adversity. These tasks are explored in a case example illustrating how these challenges reemerge across the life cycle. The key theme in this contribution is that resilience is a fluid property, a potential that practitioners and service systems can listen for, support, strengthen, and hold in trust.

Resilience has become a prominent concern for those who work with families affected by acquired brain injury (ABI). This interest can be understood to be in contrast to, even to rebuke, the focus on family burden and stress that has long been present in the ABI literature. Although this revised focus is to be welcomed, it is the view of the authors that a respectful conceptualization of resilience needs to remain sensitive to the enduring dimensions of trauma, loss, and the stress associated with brain injury. However resilient a family might be, it is never "all good" as changes post-ABI affect families in an ongoing way across the life span. Perhaps, as Higgins (1994) concluded, a positive outcome in this context is to be "struggling well"—an outcome that is an aggregate of hopefulness and strength, anguish and difficulty.

We argue the importance of maintaining a systemic and dynamic view of resilience. This systemic view has two key elements. First, there is a positive role played by support systems in catalyzing and bringing forth the inherent capacity of families to be resilient and adaptive. Second, the presence of an ABI in a family member complicates family life cycle transition points. These normative transitions, ordinarily stressful and prone to crisis, are compounded by the nonnormative adjustments that need to be made post-ABI. It is argued that assisting families attend to these extra, and quite specific, family adaptation tasks can enable practitioners and service systems to actively engage with families in ways that promote processes that build resilience.

The authors are members of a systemically oriented team that has been working with individuals and families in the ABI context for more than 20 years. Over this period of dedicated practice-based research, the team has consulted broadly, published their work, and continually reviewed and remodeled their approach to practice. What follows is an outline of the team's practice framework as applied to the concept of family resilience. This framework is illustrated by way of a case discussion. The title of the article, "Holding Resilience in Trust," speaks to the idea that resilience is not always best understood as a stable individual or family trait. Rather, resilience can be conceptualized as a dynamic and emergent quality that practitioners can listen for, strengthen, and bring forth, in the context of assisting families to negotiate key adaptation tasks following brain injury. A brief outline of the relevant literature follows. Initially, orienting information about the demography and impact of ABI is set out. Second, the emerging literature concerned with families is introduced. Finally, the subject of resilience is discussed.

The impact of ABI

ABI is common. According to the Australian Bureau of Statistics (ABS, 2003) Survey of Disability, Ageing and Carers, 1 in 45 Australians (432,700 people) had an ABI with activity limitations or participation restrictions due to disability. The impact for the individual is complex, often long term, and could include physical, cognitive, emotional, and behavioral impairments. These sequelae could result in problematic behavior for 10 to 15 years after brain injury (Brooks, Campsie, Symington, Beattie, & McKinlay, 1987; Rappaport, Herrero-Backe, Rappaport, & Winterfield, 1989; Verhaeghe, Defloor, & Grypdonck, 2005). Due to the devastating impact on daily functioning, most people with a brain injury return home and are supported primarily by family members over their lifetime (Kitter & Sharman, 2015; Zasler, Katz, Zafonte, & Arciniegas, 2012). The profound and long-lasting impact of ABI on families has been well documented in the literature spanning more than 30 years. Lezak (1988) noted that although ABI is an individual injury, it is a family affair. The high levels of distress and risks to primary and secondary caregivers associated with the trauma, psychological and behavioral changes, and burden of care are recognized. Researchers report high rates of marital separation and family distress, family breakdown, social isolation, and deterioration in health in caregivers, including high rates of anxiety and depression (Butera-Prinzi & Perlesz, 2004; Carnes & Quinn, 2005; Charles, Butera-Prinzi, & Perlesz, 2007; Eriksson, Tham, & Fugl-Meyer, 2005; Perlesz, Kinsella, & Crowe, 2000; Ponsford, Olver, Ponsford, & Nelms, 2003).

Studies indicate a clear relationship between the behavioral and emotional impairments of the individual and levels of distress and burden in families. However, acute and rehabilitation settings remain largely focused on maximizing physical and cognitive recovery for the individual with the ABI. Godwin, Lukow, and Lichiello (2015) made this point strongly when they stated that interventions that focus on the individual alone and on a medical care model are "at best inadequate and at worst ineffective" (p. 349). We argue further that a systemic and family adaptation framework is required at all stages of recovery from acute to rehabilitation and community integration, so that families can receive the care they need to mobilize emotional and physical resources to confront the difficult and unpredictable journey ahead.

Increasingly, studies are examining the effect of caregivers' well-being and functioning on outcomes for the person with ABI, further building an evidence base for the importance of family-focused work. Vangel, Rapport, and Hanks (2011), for example, examined the reciprocal influence of caregiver perceived social support and well-being in traumatic brain injury (TBI) participants in 109 pairs of TBI participants and their caregivers. Their research suggested that the strongest individual predictor of emotional distress for persons with TBI was life satisfaction of the caregiver, with the authors concluding that "interventions to promote family wellbeing may influence the wellbeing of the person with brain injury in functional, measurable ways" (Vangel et al., 2011, p. 28). Other factors found to moderate the devastating effects of TBI on survivors and family members have included social support from both professionals and peers through support groups, acceptance that life will never be the same, positive thinking and affect, spirituality, providing structure, carer management strategies, brain-injury-specific family intervention, and psychoeducation (Calvete & de Arroyabe, 2012; El Masry, Mullan, & Hackett, 2013; Elliott et al., 2015; Kitter & Sharman, 2015; Kreutzer, Marwitz, Godwin, & Arango-Lasprilla, 2010; Oddy & Herbert, 2003; Rodgers et al., 2007; Simpson & Jones, 2013). These research findings are consistent with our clinical experience with families seeking our family therapy service (Butera-Prinzi, Charles, Heine, Rutherford, & Lattin, 2009; Charles et al., 2007).

The subject of resilience

It is with an understanding of the preceding literature that the interest in resilience has emerged, mindful that the construct of family resilience has far less of a public profile and research base than does resilience as it relates to individuals. In brief, resilience can be considered as a trait characteristic—like height or temperament—or it can be conceptualized as a situational, context-dependent quality.

In so far as the latter is preferred, it follows that resilience potentially exists in all people and can be, more or less, nurtured and brought forth through responding sensitively to people's needs. Resilience, much like Saleebey's (2006) concept of strengths, is considered by the team as a dynamic and changing process in families that is shaped and influenced by the wider context, rather than a "fixed" quality or trait within individuals or the family unit. As stated by Walsh (1998), resilience is in fact developed or strengthened through experiences and interdependence with others such as family and the extended community. Family system and wider social networks can be mobilized and are "natural shock absorbers in times of crisis" (Walsh, 1998, p. 104).

In our view, families do not reach a point of resilience, or possess a steady quantum of resilience. Rather, resilience has fluidity and is influenced by many factors over the family life cycle. A family's ability to cope will vary over time depending on the circumstances and stresses being confronted and the individual, family, and community resources available at that time. Unlike individual resilience, which is often associated with personality traits or one's ability to access resources and supports, family resilience is seen as more complex and a "dynamic within the family and the networks and communities around a family that may help or hinder all individuals within the unit to cope with major difficulties and stress" (Power et al., 2016, p. 2). Hammond's definition of resilience also offers a dynamic view and emphasizes "the capacity of individuals, families, groups and community to understand and creatively draw upon their internal and external strengths, resulting in effective coping with challenges and significant adversity in ways that promote health, wellness and an increased ability to respond constructively to future adversity" (Hammond, 2008).

Higgins's (1994) notion of families "struggling well" speaks to our experience with families in our clinical setting. Families who are coping with often significant injury in their loved one, profound distress, and suffering confront these challenges with courage and determination. As underlined by Walsh (1998), those who struggle are not necessarily deficient, weak, or blameworthy, but are managing under very difficult circumstances influenced by genuine hardship (e.g., poverty, war, violence, or lack of adequate resources and social supports). For family members struggling with the aftermath of brain injury, resilience and vulnerability could coexist and sit side by side or one might be more prominent at various points in time. Masten (1994) stated that resilience needs to be understood as an interplay between particular characteristics of the individual and the broader environment, a balance between stress and the ability to cope, and a dynamic and developmental process that is important at various life transitions. Individuals could be strengthened or more vulnerable depending on the life circumstances at the time and the availability of protective factors.

Decades of research on individual and family resilience identify three dominant areas of family functioning that strengthen family capacity to navigate through times of crises and distress. These protective factors include making meaning of crisis situations and shared family belief systems, organizational structures that foster connectedness, and communication processes that are clear, consistent, and collaborative (Walsh, 2013). If families with a member with an ABI are to survive and grow through adversity, it is incumbent on health and community services to provide accessible and timely supports.

A systemic family-sensitive approach to family work post ABI

The Bouverie ABI team was established in 1983 in recognition of the complex impacts of ABI on individuals and their families. The team is funded through Disability Services, Department of Health and Human Services, and is positioned within a state-wide family therapy service and teaching institute. For the last 25 years, the team has provided a specialist brain injury family therapy service and has advocated for family-sensitive approaches to brain injury in acute, rehabilitation, and community settings through the provision of training, consultation, and postgraduate teaching in Victoria, Australia. The multidisciplinary team currently consists of one psychologist and two social workers with specialist family therapy training.

The negative effects of brain injury associated with cognitive, emotional, and behavioral changes are exacerbated or moderated through interactional patterns that develop as family members attempt, as best they can, to respond to and accommodate the effects of ABI. A systemic, family-sensitive approach is therefore required that recognizes the complex adjustments that families confront post-ABI and the crucial role systems play in providing tailored information and family-based support to facilitate these adjustments.

Guiding this approach, orienting what we do from one point to the next, are the reference points offered by the ABI Family Tasks Model that the team has developed from their work with families over several decades (Charles & Butera-Prinzi, 2008; Furlong, Young, Perlesz, McLachlan, & Riess, 1991; Perlesz, Furlong, & McLachlan, 1992; Perlesz, 1999). In this model (see Figure 1), the adjustment process post-ABI is conceptualized as involving the negotiation of four key tasks that families confront along the recovery journey. These tasks include (a) grieving and dealing with the emotional trauma of the brain injury; (b) adjusting expectations through restructuring roles and responsibilities to accommodate ABI impairments; (c) developing new identities, making meaning of what has happened, and finding value and meaning in life with an ABI; and (d) growing through adversity by developing new skills, strengths, and resources to meeting ongoing challenges.

The process of negotiating these tasks is unique to each family. It is also ongoing and shaped by particular challenges families face at different points of the family life cycle. Adjustment to ABI is thereby conceptualized as a life-long process involving the affected person, his or her immediate family, extended family, and the broader community. These tasks are conceptualized as recursively linked, in that they affect each other in reciprocal relationships.

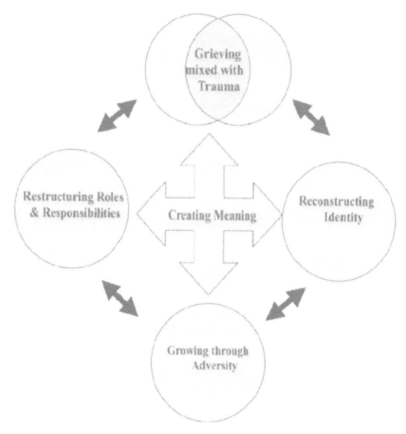

Figure 1. Family tasks model (Charles & Butera-Prinzi, 2008; Furlong et al., 1991; Perlesz, 1999; Perlesz et al., 1992).

The tasks framework helps guide conversations and interventions with families and is grounded in compassion for the difficult nature of adjustments required and in an unwavering belief in families' capacity for resilience. The holding of resilience in trust, in the face of family despair, family vulnerability, and even apparent dysfunction, helps convey messages of hope to families while acknowledging the enormity of the adjustments they face. Sometimes this requires the practitioner to hold onto hope on behalf of families during times when they appear to have lost all hope in themselves. There is no judgment, no timeline for families to meet, but rather a deep recognition and respect for each family's capacity for change and adaptation.

The team provides a counseling service that is flexible in terms of length of contact and accommodates intermittent contact over the life cycle, in recognition of the complex and changing needs of individuals and their families. Well-being and coping are promoted through fostering supportive relationships both internally, within the family, and externally, through social and community supports and connections (Butera-Prinzi et al., 2009; Butera-Prinzi, Charles, & Story, 2014; Charles & Butera-Prinzi, 2008; Charles et al., 2007).

The ABI team's integration of family therapy with peer support programs provides opportunities for families to have their experiences acknowledged and to bring forth resources, strengths, values, and goals that support family resilience. Families have drawn strength from team programs such as the Multiple Family Group Program, Tree of Life, the ABI – Family to Family Link-up Program, and the use of narrative ideas in documenting collective wisdoms that privilege skills, knowledge, and strengths from family members.

Results from these programs attest to the benefits of time-limited, facilitated, and structured programs where all family members including parents, children, siblings, and grandparents can participate. The programs acknowledge the challenges, while nurturing hope and promoting connection with others, thus reducing social isolation. Through cross-referrals and cofacilitation, the peer support programs build partnerships between ABI community agencies, offering the potential to collaboratively address the needs of family members.

In the next section, we introduce the Morris family and what brought them to counseling, followed by a description of our work with the family as guided by the ABI Family Tasks Model.

The Morris family

The referral

The Morris family consisted of Delia, age 48, her husband John, age 50, and their three children, twins Jade and Brent, age 14, and Anna, age 8. Delia sustained a severe brain injury in a motor vehicle accident at the age of 25, years before meeting her husband. Delia was in a coma for 5 weeks followed by 4 months of inpatient rehabilitation and a further 12 months of outpatient rehabilitation involving physiotherapy, speech, and occupational therapy. Although Delia had made an excellent physical recovery, she described being left with a range of cognitive difficulties including "slowed thinking, fatigue, concentration, memory, organizational skills and trouble finding the right words." At the time of the referral, the family was in crisis. Delia's husband, John, described Delia as having "disciplining issues" with the children, particularly with Jade. John said the twins often "ridiculed" their mother, because she frequently repeated herself or would say things "without thinking." John and Delia argued about differences in parenting and this was affecting their relationship. Delia felt that John undermined her parenting by criticizing her in front of the children. Delia described that John would not intervene enough with the children, leaving Delia to deal with the children's frequent arguing and fighting. John acknowledged that he could become impatient with Delia, and would intervene, at times in an angry way, which further escalated the situation.

Delia and John were desperate for help, as the situation with Jade had deteriorated to the point where she had threatened suicide and self-harm. Jade had written a desperate and poignant letter to her mother stating that she felt her only option was to run away from home, to spare her mother further grief. Mother and daughter were locked in cycles of reactivity and anger. Unfortunately, in her state of distress, Delia at times could become blaming of Jade, a response fueled by seeing her daughter as "willful" and "defiant" rather than recognizing her struggle with adolescence in the context of significant learning difficulties. John's attempts to intervene further exacerbated the difficulties as he, too, struggled with his own reactivity. Jade and Anna had both been diagnosed with learning disabilities, Jade in Grade 3 and Anna more recently. Despite Delia's efforts to get help for Jade over the years, her learning needs remained unaddressed. Delia's anxieties about her daughter's future had intensified in light of her continuing learning difficulties and were driving Delia's persistent, but unhelpful, attempts to ensure Jade kept up with her school work.

The family had previously attended Bouverie 12 years prior when the twins were 14 months old. Delia had done an extraordinary job in the context of her ABI and in managing the birth of her twins. However, her good intentions, love for her children, and determined efforts were not sufficient to override the ABI-related difficulties that affected her daily functioning. Delia's grief about her loss of capacity and vulnerability to feeling "not good enough" resurfaced in the context of becoming a mother. Delia often revisited how life would have been different had the accident not occurred. Heightened conflict between the couple regarding parenting issues settled as John came to understand Delia's anger and reactivity as a need for additional support to manage the effects of the ABI. Although contact with the Bouverie Centre ended after a few months, Delia continued to receive intensive support from her doctor, neuropsychologist, and occupational therapist with strategies to manage the demands of parenting young children and managing the household.

Although Delia had experienced John's support around her brain injury, she had also experienced being ridiculed and labeled as "backward" and "damaged" when she disclosed her ABI to extended family. After such humiliation, Delia vowed to keep her brain injury a private matter, and few people outside the immediate family knew of her brain injury. The fear of being stigmatized became a significant barrier to Delia receiving appropriate supports as the children's teachers were not aware of the additional challenges that Delia and the family faced on a daily basis.

The team's current work with the family spans a period of 2 years, with the family being seen in various combinations over 20 counseling sessions. This has included family sessions and subsystem work with the parents and separately with the children. Delia and John were also seen for individual sessions focused on trauma work. Extensive collaborative work (22 contacts) occurred with external supporting organizations involved with the family, particularly in times of crises. The number of contacts highlight the intensive work required to support families at developmentally vulnerable stages, such as negotiating the new challenges that come with young children or adolescence.

The coordinated service network

Prior to presenting an account of the therapeutic work, it is important to be clear that the team's work occurred within, and should be understood as a component of, a coordinated network response. This service network was required because the family group, and its individual members, presented multiple and complex needs in relation to which support and expertise was required from a range of health and education professionals (Keene, 2001).

Delia's general practitioner, neuropsychologist, and occupational therapist provided consistent support in the years following her brain injury and later in supporting Delia in her parenting. Team members utilized both formal (meetings) and informal consultations (regular emails and phone conversations) to work within the family's service network. This cross-agency collaboration ensured that each practitioner was aware of the roles and responsibilities of other professionals, remained clear about the family's needs and goals, was able to contain and respond effectively to the family's crises and, more generally, was able to implement the plan that had been agreed to.

Acknowledging this collaborative context as crucial, we now describe our work with the Morris family in terms of the four family tasks that families negotiate post-ABI, mindful that this is a recursive rather than a sequential process (Charles & Butera-Prinzi, 2008; Furlong et al., 1991; Perlesz, 1999; Perlesz et al., 1992).

Grieving complicated by trauma

Although the immediate concerns centered on Delia and Jade, it was apparent that all family members were involved in and affected by the escalating conflicts. Stepping back from the immediate turmoil, the team saw the family as struggling with the process of grieving. Grieving for what has been lost is always complicated for the person with the brain injury. It is also complicated for family members who know much has been lost, but remain in the presence of the person whose capacity has been changed forever. The difficulties that this context creates are now well understood, even if this issue remains diversely theorized; for example, as disenfranchised grief (Doka, 1989), putting "grief in abeyance" (Perlesz et al., 1992 p. 148), and ambiguous loss (Boss, 1991). There is no closure with grief and ABI. The challenge is for families to learn to live with the ambiguity (Boss, 1999). With the crisis involving Jade, Delia's grief about her accident, her lost potential, and thoughts about what could have been resurfaced, as they had earlier when the twins were younger. For John and the children, who had only known Delia postinjury, there was a growing awareness and compassion for what she had lost and what could have been for both Delia and the family. The grieving, for all of them, was made all the more difficult by the "invisible" nature of Delia's losses involving memory difficulties, fatigue, and problems with planning and organization.

The experience of mixed feelings is a particular feature of grief and ABI (Charles & Butera-Prinzi, 2008), and each family member is affected in a unique way and at different points in time. Delia felt both blessed to have survived the accident and have a family, and also despairing of her daily struggles to cope with brain injury. John spoke of feeling proud of Delia and all she had achieved, but at the same time feeling frustrated by her difficulties. Although adolescence brought increased capacity for Jade and Brent to better understand their mother's brain injury, it also brought the task of coming to terms with mixed feelings about her disability, further complicating their struggle with identity and independence. We saw the conflict in the family as being at least partially driven by mixed emotions and the underlying grief each family member was experiencing. Helping the family talk together about the difficulties and losses they uniquely experienced promoted growth in mutual understanding and reconnection with each other.

The presence of trauma makes an already complex grieving process even more difficult. Trauma for the individual and family members can result from traumatic memories associated with the circumstances of the injury itself, acute hospital or rehabilitation settings, or acquired impairments, including medical complications, such as seizures. In addition to this, changes in personality and behavior, particularly when marked by high levels of unpredictability, frightening behavior, or loss of trust can be conceptualized as a form of "relational trauma" involving disruption to relational bonds through the loss of trust and safety (Herman, 2001; Schore, 2009). Where grief is essentially an experience of loss, marked by sadness, trauma is marked by elevated states of anxiety, heightened stress reactions in the body, and reactivity (Charles & Butera-Prinzi, 2008).

The impact of trauma symptoms on the person with ABI and family members is increasingly being recognized in the literature (Bryant, Marosszeky, Crooks, & Gurka, 2000; Kieffer-Kristensen, Teasdale, & Bilenberg, 2011), as is the need for targeted interventions. Of critical importance is the need to compassionately but assertively respond in situations of chronic elevated conflict, and to address the potentially damaging developmental impacts on children (Beauchamp, Goodyear, von Doussa, & Young, 2013; Urbach, Sonenklar, & Culbert, 1994). The contribution of trauma for the injured person is complex due to the potential overlap between organic impacts of brain injury and posttraumatic stress disorder symptoms, involving responses such as heightened reactivity, irritability, and impacts on cognitive functioning (Bryant et al., 2000). Irrespective of the relative contribution of organic versus trauma-related factors, reducing reactivity in the person with the brain injury and in families must be prioritized for intervention.

Delia welcomed the opportunity to work individually over a series of sessions, aimed at learning calming strategies. The interventions included

(a) psychoeducation (to understand vulnerability to reactivity with ABI and trauma); (b) building body awareness skills (to recognize stress reactions in the body); (c) understanding the escalating impact of reactivity on relationships (to promote self-agency); and (d) practicing calming strategies that were accessible for Delia. Delia found the use of calming breaths and slow bilateral tapping drawn from eye movement desensitization and reprocessing (EMDR) therapy[1] particularly helpful in reducing the high levels of tension she held in her body.

The Australian Psychological Society (APS) has recently noted EMDR as a Level 1 treatment for posttraumatic stress disorder in their recent published results for "Evidence-Based Psychological Interventions: A Literature Review" (2010) for both young people and adults (available at www.Emdraa.org).

Efforts were also directed to helping Delia reframe her responses from "being a bad mother" and "a failure" to understanding her struggle as arising from a sensitive nervous system and overload of stress. This reframing helped validate her distress and good intentions as a mother. At the same time, both in individual and family therapy, we maintained a compassionate but strong line about the need for Delia to take responsibility to find ways to moderate her responses. John, as the other adult, was equally called on to take responsibility to both support Delia in her efforts and manage his own responses so as not to escalate situations further. Psychoeducation on trauma also assisted John in understanding the potential traumatic impacts of escalating arguments for children and therefore the need for John to manage his own responses. Delia would benefit from further individual work to address possible ongoing effects from the trauma of the accident itself, as well as grief associated with her injury, so as to reduce emotional factors contributing to elevated stress responses and reactivity.

Lack of community understanding of the complexities of ABI adds to the sense of social isolation and disenfranchised grief, arising from a lack of validation and social recognition of their losses. As expressed by Delia, "I look fine, so others don't understand that each day is a struggle to remember, to make sure I am organized, that I haven't forgotten something important. I get tired and need to have a sleep."

Adjusting expectations through restructuring roles and responsibilities

ABI causes impairments and changed functioning in an individual. Depending on the role this person performs in his or her family, ABI forces readjustments and sometimes radical reallocations of roles and responsibilities. Letting go of valued roles and restructuring one's life and family is profoundly difficult. There is a deep sense of loss as change is "imposed" by virtue of the ABI. Ironically, the better the person's recovery and insight, the more difficult and painful the process of letting go of previous roles and readjusting expectations can be, as the person is "so close and yet so far" from being able to function in the way he or she once did.

This process of readjusting roles (and therefore relationships) occurs in all areas of a person's life including work, leisure activities, social networks, community roles, parenting, and partnership roles. Increased responsibilities or role reversals by primary carers, generally partners or parents, or siblings and children as secondary carers, can be overwhelming, developmentally restrictive, and understandably generate feelings of resentment (Furlong et al., 1991). What can promote family members' readjustment to new expectations and lifestyle is the acknowledgment of the losses and acceptance of the permanence of the disability and the changes required (Furlong et al., 1991).

In keeping with their own family of origin and cultural experiences, Delia and John had defined roles in the family. Delia valued her identity as a "good mother" and struggled with acknowledging the impact of the brain injury on her identity and her parenting. With ongoing supports from specialist brain injury services, including her doctor, neuropsychologist, and occupational therapist, Delia had developed routines and strategies to compensate for the difficulties with short-term memory, fatigue, planning, and organization. John was the financial provider and worked long hours to ensure financial security and capacity for the family to enjoy outings and activities, which he and the family highly valued. Although these defined roles had served them well as a family with young children, adjustments of their roles were necessary with the children moving toward adolescence and naturally developing physical, emotional, and social independence.

Delia and John had different expectations of each other regarding their parenting roles. Delia was clearly seeking more support from John, particularly as she was not coping with increased protests from the children and Jade's emotional reactivity and defiance, and John was relying on Delia to manage and discipline the children. Both John and Delia brought individual vulnerabilities to dealing with conflict from their own family of origin, which in the context of adolescence, stretched the family beyond their current coping abilities.

John experienced high levels of conflict in his family of origin, which led him to leave home in late adolescence, whereas Delia avoided conflict by being compliant. John and Delia's responses to conflict oscillated between avoidance and overreacting, which inevitably drove the family into chaos. Delia's levels of stress increased sharply at times of heightened conflict or when she felt she was "losing control." She often complained of feeling confused and that her "head was going to explode." Feeling overwhelmed himself, John often criticized Delia for her "irrationality," which diminished Delia's confidence and undermined her authority as a parent. Delia often complained that "the children do not listen to me. I have no authority." Delia's strongly held wish was to forge a positive bond with her children, to be able to spend quality time and have fun with them, and in particular develop a good mother–daughter relationship with both girls. This strong desire led her to access the necessary assistance.

Work with the couple focused on ways in which Delia and John could support each other in their parenting. John made efforts to more actively participate in managing the children's conflicts and needs by assisting with issues relating to homework, access to the computer, sibling rivalry, and social outings. This enabled Delia, in turn, to be less reactive and more playful with the children as she felt less burdened and more supported as a parent. Reframing the meaning of Jade's behavior from one of defiance and "not caring" to struggling to negotiate adolescence and learning difficulties, Delia and John were able to relate to Jade with greater understanding and compassion, making room for tolerance, effective problem solving, warmth, and respect. Delia was encouraged to step back from the role of monitoring Jade's every move and take on the role of building Jade's self-esteem by sharing positive experiences and together working toward emotional regulation by remaining calm and nonreactive.

By supporting Delia to refocus her role as a mother on activities where she could experience success and pride, escalating cycles of conflict were interrupted and positive, nurturing cycles were promoted. Delia came to accept that although she could not "fix" her children's learning difficulties, she could provide her children with positive experiences and an affirming environment within the family home. Within the context of a more positive and nurturing family environment, the children were able to show more understanding and compassion toward their mother and accept greater age-appropriate responsibilities. Despite the ongoing challenges and necessary support from specialist service providers, the family was experiencing a closer, more positive connection with a calmer, less conflictual family environment that was generally happy and no longer characterized by constant screaming and yelling.

Developing new identities and meanings

In so much as respective roles and responsibilities have to be renegotiated, to this degree personal identity has to be transformed. The challenge is to incorporate changed capacities without taking on an all-encompassing identity of deficiency. Making meaning of what has happened and finding new ways to participate and contribute to family life and community facilitates identities of value that incorporate both the disability and capacities.

Delia and John were able to readjust their roles to better accommodate the challenges of adolescence and their children's learning needs. Over time, Delia grew to appreciate her skills as a mother and she no longer felt defined by the difficulties associated with the ABI. By developing new meanings of their family difficulties that were more compassionate, normalizing, and validating of strengths and capacities, Delia was able to take the step of informing the school about her ABI for the first time. Delia received validation of her efforts, courage, and persistence, particularly in the context of having two children with special learning needs. Both Delia and John were able to shift from identities associated with shame and diminished worth to ones associated with pride and strengthened faith in their own capacities and resilience. Delia's children face the task of incorporating new understandings about their mother's disability. This capacity increases over time as children's developmental capacities expand. It is crucial here that children are given accurate information about brain injuries that incorporate strengths, capacity for growth and development, as well as ABI-related difficulties.

Growing through adversity

This task involves reaching the realization that, although loss is ongoing, growth has occurred in dealing with adversity. This sense of growth is associated with recognition of the new skills, strengths, and resources that have been developed in meeting ongoing challenges and include recognizing qualities such as determination, courage, and resilience. It also involves the reexamining of one's values and priorities in life in light of the experience of sustaining a brain injury and realization of the fragility of life. Common changes include increased gratitude for what one has, deepened compassion for others, changed priorities, and valuing the present.

Delia and John were determined to stay together and work toward their desired goals of reduced conflict and improved family well-being. Counseling provided a space where their shared values could be acknowledged and highlighted. Inviting family members to reflect on the skills and strengths that emerged through their struggles transformed their relationships with each other.

The following factors were supported through the counseling process, enabling the family to experience a sense of growth and increased capacity for resilience in the face of ongoing challenges.

Delia and John's shared value of commitment toward the family unit and balancing family connectedness with individual needs

This was demonstrated by Delia's encouragement of the children participating in preparing and sharing evening meals. John showed a keen interest in regular planned family outings that provided the children with new experiences and gave the family an opportunity to have fun together. Delia and John worked toward increasing mutual respect, being equal partners, and providing cooperative parenting and caregiving. This served to strengthen the couple's relationship and provide family stability and continuity in the face of family stresses. With a clear and united leadership, the children were less reactive and showed greater care for each other, leading to improved family functioning.

The family's ability to gain a shared and relational view of their struggles and strengths increased family cohesiveness, connectedness, and hope. As family members gained a greater appreciation and acceptance of the limitations that come with ABI and learning disabilities, their responses shifted from personal attacks and criticism to noticing individual good intentions and achievements. The family became more adept at punctuating challenging moments with positive affirmations, resulting in family members being more compassionate, tolerant, and supportive toward each other. Normalizing Jade and Brent's rebellious behavior as natural adolescent behavior rather than intentionally disruptive or belligerent assisted Delia and John in remaining sensitive and flexible in their parenting style and gaining an increased appreciation of Jade and Brent's skills and growing independence. The consequent reduction in reactivity increased the family's engagement in pleasurable activities and provided a welcome respite from difficult times.

Positive mediating environmental influences were equally powerful in lessening vulnerability

Important factors included strong mentoring relationships with church and youth groups with whom the family had a strong sense of belonging; kin networks, namely extended family and friends who Delia could use as respite when feeling overwhelmed or distressed; and increased communication and a working alliance with school personnel to address Jade and Anna's special learning needs. The consistent involvement and collaboration with specialist health professionals provided a sense of safety and security the family could rely on without being judged or blamed. Although Delia's cognitive impairments are permanent, a focus on her abilities, values, and goals proved far more effective in overcoming the challenges. Compensatory strategies were implemented so that she could work toward improved communication and problem solving and successfully manage a busy household while attending to both her needs and the needs of each family member. These factors align with the research findings of Walsh (2013) that identified shared family beliefs and meaning making, family organization, structure and connectedness, and communication as key protective processes that promote family resilience.

Discussion

This account of our work with the Morris family was designed to highlight the team's approach to practice. In this approach, an ABI is considered a major "nonnormative" complication in terms of family life cycle development where, over time, the larger challenge for families is to find a way to accommodate to this event within the context of the family negotiating their normative developmental demands (Carter & McGoldrick, 1998). The potentially negative impacts of ABI are exacerbated at points of life cycle transitions, where families need to adapt and change to meet new developmental needs. At these points of change, stress is often heightened for these families, due to complications caused by ABI-related difficulties such as memory impairments, fatigue, and emotional reactivity. For the Morris family, this occurred at the point of transition to new parenthood and then 12 years later, when adjusting to adolescence.

Despite occasions of emotional and behavioral crisis, potential strengths remain, and can be activated, if these episodes can be contained and practically responded to, and if practitioners can keep the family's resilience "in trust" despite the intense feelings that can be expressed. Containing the sense of crisis that is often present can be challenging, but is essential if the practitioner is not to inadvertently align with the loss of hope that can occur in times of crisis. In taking up this orientation, practitioners need to be mindful of, and active in relation to, family-system issues such as the importance of mobilizing timely environmental supports.

By holding resilience "in trust," families and practitioners alike can remain connected to family strengths and potential for growth and change in the midst of difficulties. Working toward family resilience involves many interactive processes over time. What is helpful at one stage is not at another (Walsh, 1998). Because of the ongoing nature of challenges associated with ABI, notions of resilience need to incorporate the reworking of key family tasks that occur across the life cycle. These include working through grief and emotional trauma as it resurfaces at points of transition or in times of crisis; restructuring of roles in response to changing developmental needs in the family; reshaping of identity in the context of changed roles, new life goals, and purposes; and finally, growing through adversity involving discovery and development of new meanings, skills, and capacities through facing challenges. Despite the challenges that often come with ABI, "adversities can be transformative, yielding new life, priorities, purpose, and positive growth" (Walsh, 2013, p. 72).

With ABI, resilience is present and co-occurs in the context of expressions of grief at loss of capacity, frustrations of living with ABI-related impairments, and the ongoing challenge of incorporating disability into one's identity while maintaining a sense of worth, value, and capacity. As such, resilience is not a fixed quality, not a process of bouncing back or an end state to be reached, but rather a dynamic and changing process that often coexists with continuing struggles. Over our 25 years of practice, we have been inspired by the courage with which these families face the ongoing challenges. Importantly, resilience is relational and systemic, arising in the context of relationships with others, within the family and within broader support systems.

Families affected by ABI need affirmation of their strength and courage as they can easily fall vulnerable to a sense of shame, blame, guilt, and worthlessness brought about by the enduring challenges of ABI. Rather than pathologizing their actions and responses, families need reminding of the extraordinary job they are doing in the context of what they are dealing with, their inherent worth as human beings, and our unwavering faith, as practitioners, in their capacity to deal with challenges, given appropriate supports and assistance. The challenge as practitioners is to maintain our efforts to tailor our responses to address specific family needs as best we can, albeit within systems often lacking adequate resources to address the complexity of what is required. Alongside holding both hope and despair with families, practitioners are required to "change the odds against them" (Walsh, 1998,

p. 12) through the active implementation and resourcing of effective family programs and social support systems. This article has outlined our approach to resilience and illustrated through a case study how timely intervention focused on assisting families to navigate ABI adaptational tasks in the context of new developmental challenges can change family dynamics and mobilize family capacities toward increasing resilience. Practitioners and service providers play a critical role in bringing forth the inherent capacities of all families to adapt and cope with the challenges that come with ABI.

Note

1. Unlike the death of a loved one where there is a clear loss and mourning, with ambiguous loss there is no closure as the person may be alive but psychologically or cognitively unavailable as in dementia or acquired brain injury.

Acknowledgments

Our thanks to the Morris family for their permission to draw on their experience in this article. We would also like to thank Dr. Mark Furlong, Thinker in Residence, Adjunct Senior Lecturer, The Bouverie Centre, for his assistance in preparing this material.

References

Australian Institute of Health and Welfare. (2007). *Disability in Australia: Acquired brain injury.* Canberra, Australia: AIHW.

Beauchamp, J., Goodyear, M., von Doussa, H., & Young, J. (2013). *Child aware approaches project: Trauma-informed family sensitive practice for adult oriented health services.*

Guidelines for trauma informed family sensitive practice in adult health services. Melbourne, Australia: The Bouverie Centre.

Boss, P. (1991). *Living beyond loss: Death in the family*. New York, NY: Norton.

Boss, P. (1999). *Ambiguous loss: Learning to live with unresolved grief*. London, UK: Harvard University Press.

Brooks, N., Campsie, L., Symington, C., Beattie, A., & McKinlay, W. (1987). The effects of severe head injury on patient and relatives within seven years of injury. *The Journal of Head Trauma Rehabilitation, 2*(3), 1–13. doi:10.1097/00001199-198709000-00003

Bryant, R. A., Marosszeky, J. E., Crooks, J., & Gurka, J. (2000). Posttraumatic stress disorder after severe traumatic brain injury. *American Journal of Psychiatry, 157*, 629–631. doi:10.1176/appi.ajp.157.4.629

Butera-Prinzi, F., Charles, N., Heine, K., Rutherford, B., & Lattin, D. (2009). Family-to-family link up program: A community-based initiative supporting families caring for someone with an acquired brain injury. *NeuroRehabilitation, 27*(1), 31–47.

Butera-Prinzi, F., Charles, N., & Story, K. (2014). Narrative family therapy and group work for families living with acquired brain injury. *Australian and New Zealand Journal of Family Therapy, 35*(1), 81–99. doi:10.1002/anzf.1046

Butera-Prinzi, F., & Perlesz, A. (2004). Through children's eyes: Children's experience of living with a parent with an acquired brain injury. *Brain Injury, 18*, 83–101. doi:10.1080/02699050310001185 00

Calvete, E., & de Arroyabe, E. L. (2012). Depression and grief in Spanish family caregivers of people with traumatic brain injury: The roles of social support and coping. *Brain Injury, 26*, 834–843. doi:10.3109/02699052.2012.655363

Carnes, S. L., & Quinn, W. H. (2005). Family adaptation to brain injury: Coping and psychological distress. *Families, Systems, & Health, 23*, 186–203. doi:10.1037/1091-7527.23.2.186

Carter, B., & McGoldrick, M. (1998). *The expanded family life cycle: Individual, family, and social perspectives* (3rd ed.). Needham Hill, MA: Allyn & Bacon.

Charles, N., & Butera-Prinzi, F. (2008). Acquired brain injury: Reconstructing meaning following traumatic grief. *Grief Matters, 11*, 64–69.

Charles, N., Butera-Prinzi, F., & Perlesz, A. (2007). Families living with acquired brain injury: A multiple family group experience. *NeuroRehabilitation, 22*(1), 61–76.

Doka, K. (1989). *Disenfranchised grief: Recognizing hidden sorrow*. Lexington, MA: D. C. Heath.

El Masry, Y., Mullan, B., & Hackett, M. (2013). Psychosocial experiences and needs of Australian caregivers of people with stroke: Prognosis messages, caregiver resilience, and relationships. *Topics in Stroke Rehabilitation, 20*, 356–368. doi:10.1310/tsr2004-356

Elliott, T. R., Hsiao, Y. Y., Kimbrel, N. A., Meyer, E. C., DeBeer, B. B., Gulliver, S. B., & Morissette, S. B. (2015). Resilience, traumatic brain injury, depression, and posttraumatic stress among Iraq/Afghanistan war veterans. *Rehabilitation Psychology, 60*, 263–276. doi:10.1037/rep0000050

Eriksson, G., Tham, K., & Fugl-Meyer, A. R. (2005). Couples' happiness and its relationship to functioning in everyday life after brain injury. *Scandinavian Journal of Occupational Therapy, 12*(1), 40–48. doi:10.1080/11038120510027630

Furlong, M., Young, J., Perlesz, A., McLachlan, D., & Riess, C. (1991). For family therapists involved in the treatment of chronic and longer term conditions. *Dulwich Centre Newsletter, 4*, 58–68.

Godwin, E. E., Lukow, H. R., & Lichiello, S. (2015). Promoting resilience following traumatic brain injury: Application of an interdisciplinary, evidence-based model for intervention. *Family Relations, 64*, 347–362. doi:10.1111/fare.12122

Hammond, W. (2008). *Family resilience.* Royal Mount University Research Bytes No. 3, Fall 2011. Retrieved from http://www.mtroyal.ca/cs/groups/public/documents/pdf/familyresiliencyrb.pdf

Herman, J. (2001). *Trauma and recovery: From domestic abuse to political terror.* London, UK: Pandora.

Higgins, G. O. C. (1994). *Resilient adults: Overcoming a cruel past.* San Francisco, CA: Jossey-Bass.

Keene, J. (2001). *Clients with complex needs: Inter-professional practice.* Oxford, UK: Blackwell Science.

Kieffer-Kristensen, R., Teasdale, T. W., & Bilenberg, N. (2011). Post-traumatic stress symptoms and psychological functioning in children of parents with acquired brain injury. *Brain Injury, 25,* 752–760. doi:10.3109/02699052.2011.579933

Kitter, B., & Sharman, R. (2015). Caregivers' support needs and factors promoting resiliency after brain injury. *Brain Injury, 29,* 1082–1093. doi:10.3109/02699052.2015.1018323

Kreutzer, J. S., Marwitz, J. H., Godwin, E. E., & Arango-Lasprilla, J. C. (2010). Practical approaches to effective family intervention after brain injury. *The Journal of Head Trauma Rehabilitation, 25,* 113–120. doi:10.1097/htr.0b013e3181cf0712

Lezak, M. D. (1988). Brain damage is a family affair. *Journal of Clinical and Experimental Neuropsychology, 10*(1), 111–123. doi:10.1080/01688638808405098

Masten, A. (1994). Resilience in individual development: Successful adaptation despite risk and adversity. In M. C. Wang & E. W. Gordon (Eds.), *Educational resilience in inner-city America: Challenges and prospects* (pp. 3–25). Hillsdale, NJ: Erlbaum.

Oddy, M., & Herbert, C. (2003). Intervention with families following brain injury: Evidence-based practice. *Neuropsychological Rehabilitation, 13*(1–2), 259–273. doi:10.1080/09602010244000345

Perlesz, A. (1999). Complex responses to trauma: Challenges in bearing witness. *Australian and New Zealand Journal of Family Therapy, 20*(1), 11–19. doi:10.1111/j.0814-723x.1999.00089.x

Perlesz, A., Furlong, M., & McLachlan, D. (1992). Family work and acquired brain damage. *Australian and New Zealand Journal of Family Therapy, 13,* 145–153. doi:10.1002/j.1467-8438.1992.tb00910.x

Perlesz, A., Kinsella, G., & Crowe, S. (2000). Psychological distress and family satisfaction following traumatic brain injury: Injured individuals and their primary, secondary, and tertiary carers. *The Journal of Head Trauma Rehabilitation, 15,* 909–929. doi:10.1097/00001199-200006000-00005

Ponsford, J., Olver, J., Ponsford, M., & Nelms, R. (2003). Long-term adjustment of families following traumatic brain injury where comprehensive rehabilitation has been provided. *Brain Injury, 17,* 453–468. doi:10.1080/0269905031000070143

Power, J., Goodyear, M., Maybery, D., Reupert, A., O'Hanlon, B., Cuff, R., & Perlesz, A. (2016). Family resilience in families where a parent has a mental illness. *Journal of Social Work, 16*(1), 66–82. doi:10.1177/1468017314568081

Rappaport, M., Herrero-Backe, C., Rappaport, M. L., & Winterfield, K. M. (1989). Head injury outcome up to ten years later. *Archives of Physical Medicine and Rehabilitation, 70,* 885–892.

Rodgers, M. L., Strode, A. D., Norell, D. M., Short, R. A., Dyck, D. G., & Becker, B. (2007). Adapting multiple-family group treatment for brain and spinal cord injury intervention development and preliminary outcomes. *American Journal of Physical Medicine & Rehabilitation, 86,* 482–492. doi:10.1097/phm.0b013e31805c00a1

Saleebey, D. (2006). *The strengths perspective in social work practice.* Boston, MA: Pearson/Allyn & Bacon.

Schore, A. N. (2009). Relational trauma and the developing right brain. *Annals of the New York Academy of Sciences, 1159*(1), 189–203. doi:10.1111/j.1749-6632.2009.04474.x

Simpson, G., & Jones, K. (2013). How important is resilience among family members supporting relatives with traumatic brain injury or spinal cord injury? *Clinical Rehabilitation, 27,* 367–377. doi:10.1177/0269215512457961

Urbach, J. R., Sonenklar, N., & Culbert, J. (1994). Risk factors and assessment in children of brain-injured parents. *Journal of Neuropsychiatry, 6,* 289–295. doi:10.1176/jnp.6.3.289

Vangel, S. J., Jr., Rapport, L. J., & Hanks, R. A. (2011). Effects of family and caregiver psychosocial functioning on outcomes in persons with traumatic brain injury. *The Journal of Head Trauma Rehabilitation, 26*(1), 20–29. doi:10.1097/htr.0b013e318204a70d

Verhaeghe, S., Defloor, T., & Grypdonck, M. (2005). Stress and coping among families of patients with traumatic brain injury: A review of the literature. *Journal of Clinical Nursing, 14,* 1004–1012. doi:10.1111/j.1365-2702.2005.01126.x

Walsh, F. (1998). *Strengthening family resilience.* New York, NY: Guilford.

Walsh, F. (2013). Community-based practice application of a family resilience framework. In D. S. Becvar (Ed.), *Handbook of family resilience* (pp. 65–82). New York, NY: Springer.

Zasler, N. D., Katz, D. I., Zafonte, R. D., & Arciniegas, D. B. (Eds.). (2012). *Brain injury medicine: Principles and practice.* New York, NY: Demos Medical.

Brain Injury as the Result of Violence: A Systematic Scoping Review

Annerley Bates, Sarah Matthews, Grahame Simpson, and Lyndel Bates

ABSTRACT

This scoping review investigated risk factors, impacts, outcomes, and service implications of violence-related traumatic brain injury (TBI) for individuals and their informal caregivers. A systematic search (Web of Science, PubMed, PsycInfo, ProQuest, Medline, Informit; 1990–2015) identified 17 studies meeting the inclusion and exclusion criteria. Violence was the cause of between 3% and 26% of all TBIs. Males, a non-White racial background, preinjury unemployment, and preinjury substance abuse problems all elevated the risk for sustaining a violence-related TBI compared to other-cause TBI. However, few differences were observed in 12 months postinjury outcomes. No studies investigated the impact of violence-related TBI on informal caregivers.

Violence is an international public health issue resulting in premature death, disability, and injury (Krug, Dahlberg, Mercy, Zwi, & Lozano, 2002) with as many as 14,249 deaths in the United States reported as arising from violence (Federal Bureau of Investigation, 2014). In Australia, violence is also an issue of national concern, with extensive media coverage of violence that results in the death of a person (e.g., Atkinson, 2014; Berg, 2014; Dow, 2013; Farrow, 2015). Additionally, it has been estimated that for each death by violence, there are 100 nonfatal violence-related injuries (Rosenberg & Fenley, 1991).

Traumatic brain injury (TBI) is one type of injury that can result from violence (Faul, Xu, Wald, & Coronado, 2010). TBI is a leading cause of disability globally (World Health Organization [WHO] Global Consultation on Violence and Health, 1996). A TBI can be defined as an injury to brain tissue that has occurred due to an external force resulting in marked cognitive, social, behavioral, and physical changes that affect the individual and his or her family (Arango-Lasprilla et al., 2008; Harrison-Felix et al., 1998). The most common causes of TBI are motor vehicle crashes, falls, sporting injuries, and violence-related mechanisms (Simpson, Simons, & McFadyen, 2002).

In the most recent research regarding violence-related TBI, investigators have broadly characterized violence as arising from physical assault or gunshot (Gerhart, Mellick, & Weintraub, 2003; Hanlon, Demery, Martinovich, & Kelly, 1999; Harrison-Felix et al., 1998; Kim, Colantonio, Bayley, & Dawson, 2011; Machamer, Temkin, & Dikmen, 2003; Schopp, Good, Barker, Mazurek, & Hathaway, 2006; Wenden, Crawford, Wade, King, & Moss, 1998). Although intentionality can be difficult to determine because it infers a state of mind, the construct of other-inflicted (harm caused by others) versus self-inflicted (harm caused by oneself) is also incorporated into definitions (Gerhart et al., 2003; Harrison-Felix et al., 1998; Kim & Colantonio, 2008; Kim et al., 2011; Schopp et al., 2006; Wagner, Sasser, Hammond, Wiercisieswski, & Alexander, 2000). In general, the approach within these studies is consistent with the WHO Global Consultation on Violence and Health (1996) definition of violence as "the intentional use of physical force or power, threatened or actual, against oneself, another person, or against a group or a community, that either results in or has a high likelihood of resulting in injury, death, psychological harm, mal-development or deprivation" (p. 3).

Research into violence-related TBI found that there are a significant minority of individuals sustaining an injury as a result of violence. In the United States, physical assault accounted for 10% of all brain injuries from 2002 to 2006, with 21% of the most severe injuries requiring medical attention and hospitalization (Faul et al., 2010). Canada reports that 8% to 10% of hospital admissions are the result of physical assault (Colantonio et al., 2010; Kim & Colantonio, 2008), whereas in Australia in 2004 and 2005, 16.8% of hospital admissions for TBI were the result of an assault (Helps, Henley, & Harrison, 2008). A range of significant impacts has been reported on individuals sustaining violence-related TBI including persisting neurological symptoms, neuropsychological impairments, and poor psychosocial outcomes (Gerhart et al., 2003; Harrison-Felix et al., 1998; Machamer et al., 2003).

Families also face significant disruption when a relative sustains a TBI from any cause including violence. This includes experiencing elevated levels of depression and anxiety, carer burden, increased health-seeking behavior, reductions in employment, and changes in family functioning and roles (Anderson, Simpson, & Morey, 2013; Boycott, Yeoman, & Vesey, 2013; Degeneffe, 2001; Hall et al., 1994; Ponsford, Olver, Ponsford, & Nelms, 2003). Research among other populations has found that vicarious strain can occur when the family or informal caregiver is a direct witness to the violence, hears the violence occurring, or hears about the violence. In particular, violent crime victims (including assault) and their families are at greater risk of developing post-traumatic stress disorder (Freedy, Resnick, Kilpatrick, Danksy, & Tidwell, 1994) and it is important to ascertain whether the same experience has been documented in families supporting relatives with violence-related TBI.

People who sustain violence-related TBIs might also experience challenges and disadvantage in navigating service systems to access needed rehabilitation and longer term support services (Esselman, Dikmen, Bell, & Temkin, 2004). Additionally, the families who play a vital role in progressing the rehabilitation of their relative (Elbaum, 2007) might have to navigate both the health and the criminal justice systems. Complicating this challenge, family members or informal caregivers might not be included in decisions and actions taken by hospitals, with one study suggesting that families are not routinely involved by staff in emergency departments for all patients who are admitted due to violence (Linnarsson, Benzein, & Arestedt, 2014).

The issue of violence-related TBI is of substantial significance. In addition to the extensive range of impacts experienced by the person and his or her family members, at a macrolevel, the financial costs to society of violence-related TBI are significant. There are the direct costs of acute medical care and rehabilitation, as well as indirect costs through the ongoing care, support services, loss of an individual's productivity, and the administration of health insurance and disability payments to individuals (Caro, 2011; Finkelstein, Corso, & Miller, 2006; Harrison-Felix et al., 1998). The estimated lifetime cost of a severe TBI in Australia is $4.8 million per person (Picenna, Pattuwage, Gruen, & Bragge, 2014) so accordingly, TBIs could represent one of the most expensive outcomes of assault. In fact, Helps et al. (2008) estimated that the direct hospital cost of assault-related TBIs in Australia is $15.7 million per annum.

Despite the importance of the topic, to the best of our knowledge, there has not yet been a systematic review of the research in this area. Given the lack of previous reviews, a scoping approach was selected, as it is a well-suited methodology to identify the breadth and depth of evidence within a defined field, particular in areas where the research evidence might be limited, heterogeneous, or fragmented (Levac, Colquhoun, & O'Brien, 2010). The research question was this: What are the risk factors, impacts, outcomes, and service implications of violence-related TBI for individuals and informal caregivers? By answering this research question, researchers and policymakers will be able to develop and implement interventions targeted at this particular subpopulation of injured persons.

Method

The scoping review used the five stages originally outlined by Arksey and O'Malley (2005) and later refined by Levac et al. (2010). The stages are (a) identifying the research question, (b) identifying relevant studies, (c) study selection, (d) charting the data, and (e) collating, summarizing, and reporting results.

Identifying the research question

To identify the research question, the concept, target population, and health outcome of interest were defined to clearly articulate the scope of enquiry (Levac et al., 2010). The construct of violence within research specifically applied to sustaining a TBI in a civilian context as the result of intentional force arising from gunshot or physical assault. Therefore, it did not encompass studies that considered other dimensions of violence such as threatened violence, or violence targeting families, groups, or communities. Research regarding TBI that occurred in a military conflict setting was excluded, as personnel from this context were more likely to present with a range of comorbidities associated with being involved in warfare; this presents unique rehabilitation and caregiving needs that are likely to influence the psychosocial outcomes of individuals and informal caregivers of this population (Burke, Degeneffe, & Olney, 2009). The review was international in scope.

The target population was adults who were the victims of the violence, as well as their families and informal caregivers. People sustaining violence-related pediatric brain injury were not included in the study. The term *informal caregiver* was defined as a nonprofessional provider of care to a person with violence-related TBI; formal caregivers such as nurses and allied health workers were excluded. Health outcomes of interest included predisposing risk factors (i.e., demographic and psychosocial variables), injury-related factors (e.g., severity of TBI, other injuries associated with polytrauma), outcomes (e.g., presence of symptoms, impairments, functional status, social reintegration), service pathways and costs (e.g., accessing inpatient rehabilitation, health costs payer), and family well-being and relationship stability.

Identifying relevant studies

A two-step search strategy was employed. First, a systematic search was conducted employing a number of electronic databases and search engines: Web of Science, PubMed, PsycInfo, ProQuest, Medline, and Informit. These are common databases used for the conduct of literature reviews within the field of TBI, capturing all the key journals in the health and rehabilitation fields. Search terms were identified by reviewing the literature that discussed individual family and caregiver psychosocial outcomes in a TBI setting and selecting keywords that were relevant to the research question. Search terms were grouped according to population characteristics (family, informal caregivers, TBI, violence) and health outcomes (psychosocial adjustment, family functioning, and navigating systems). Multiple overlapping terms were used to give the best possible scope of studies identified in the search (see Table 1). Limiting functions were applied to select human studies and articles published in English. The second stage involved hand-searching reference lists from studies identified through the initial electronic search to identify any further works.

Study selection

Studies were selected if (a) they contained original research on TBI resulting from violence, (b) the study variables were compared to people who sustained

Table 1. Search strategy.

Population	
Informal caregivers	"carer*" OR "caregiver*" OR "caregiving" OR "family caregiving" OR "family" OR "families" OR "informal caregivers"
	AND
TBI	"traumatic brain injury" OR "TBI" OR "head injury" OR "brain injury" OR "brain injuries" OR "severe brain injury" OR "brain damage" OR "craniocerebral trauma"
	AND
Violence	"violence" OR "assault" OR "physical assault" OR "violent crime" OR "aggression" OR "aggressive behavior" OR "criminal justice system" OR "intentional injury"
	AND
	Health Outcomes
Psychosocial adjustment	"psychosocial adjust*" OR "quality of life" OR "mental health" OR "coping" OR "life satisfaction" OR "stress" OR "depression" OR "anxiety" OR "psychological" OR "burnout" OR "vicarious trauma" OR "depressive symptom*" OR "depressive disorder*" OR "satisfaction with life" OR "SWL" OR "caregiver burden*" OR "psychological distress" OR "caregiver distress" OR "QOL" OR "drugs" OR "alcohol" OR "self medication" OR "self-medication"
	OR
Family functioning	"family functioning" OR "family needs" OR "family adjustment" OR "family system" OR "family breakdown" OR "family engagement" OR "family structure" OR "spouse*" OR "sibling*" OR "parent*"
	OR
Navigating systems	"support system*" OR "services" OR "social support" OR "criminal justice system" OR "health system" OR "legal system" OR "service system" OR "non-government organi*ation" OR "NGO" OR "civil societ*" OR "police" OR "police officers" OR "hospital" OR "emergency" OR "rehabilitation unit" OR "social worker*" OR "psychologist*" OR "allied health" OR "lawyer*" OR "neuropsychiatrist*" OR "neuropsychologist*" OR "psychiatrist*" OR "accessibility" OR "community support" OR "patient caregiver advocate"

Note: An asterisk (*) indicates a truncated word as part of the search. SWL = satisfaction with Life; QOL = quality of Life; NGO = nongovernmental organization.

TBI from other causes, and (c) the comparisons were tested statistically. Studies were excluded if (a) they were non-peer-reviewed citations (e.g., unpublished dissertations, abstracts, conference proceedings, books, commentary, and editorials), and (b) if the study population was not clearly defined as including TBI resulting from violence. Given the limited number of papers that only included individuals with violence-related TBIs, studies were incorporated if they considered this group as a subpopulation within their wider research.

The database search results were entered into an EndNote library database, which was then used to identify and remove duplicates. Screening occurred in two stages. Initially, two authors (Sarah Matthews and Lyndel Bates) examined the titles and abstracts of the citations individually against the inclusion and exclusion criteria and then compared their individual results. The identified studies then underwent a second stage of screening where full-text articles were read (Sarah Matthews) to determine if the full inclusion criteria were met. During this stage additional articles were identified by reviewing the reference lists. The articles retained after this stage were then read by all authors and a final decision about inclusion was made by consensus.

Data charting

Several templates were devised that would allow identification of data that were relevant to the research question. The first involved collecting descriptive data to characterize all the studies identified in the search including first author, year of publication, country where the research was conducted, study design, service setting and source of the data, the definition of violence used, sample size and time since injury, etiology and breakdown, and measures used. A further five templates were devised to collect data on the five review questions, namely premorbid and demographic features, injury and injury-related factors, outcomes, service pathways and costs, and caregiver outcomes. The specific data fields for each question are specified in the Results.

Collating, summarizing, and reporting results

Given the broad heterogeneity of studies and variables, a qualitative rather than quantitative (i.e., meta-analytic) synthesis was conducted, seeking to identify patterns and commonalities in the research findings across participants (individual, formal caregiver, or both), settings, outcomes, and service pathways (for a discussion of the difference between quantitative and qualitative synthesis, see Carter, Lubinsky & Domholdt, 2011; for another example of the qualitative synthesis of findings from quantitative studies, see Wheeler, Accord-Vira, & Davis, 2016). This approach is different to reviews that undertake thematic synthesis of qualitative research (e.g., Thomas & Harden, 2008).

Citations were grouped into studies focusing on the individual and studies with data relating to families. Six tables were then constructed to tabulate the data from the templates. Given the large number of findings reported for some of the review variables, only findings that exceeded a more stringent p value of .01 were reported. This also helped address the problem that some studies reported results from multiple univariate statistical tests without controlling for possible Type II error.

Results

The search terms retrieved a total of 569 articles from the database search (see Figure 1). Titles and associated details were compiled into an EndNote database where 214 duplicates were identified and removed. The remaining abstracts were then screened to identify those potential articles that met the inclusion criteria. A total of 44 full-text articles were identified at this stage. Review of these articles' list of references identified further articles for inclusion. The selected articles were then reviewed against the inclusion and exclusion criteria, with 17 being retained.

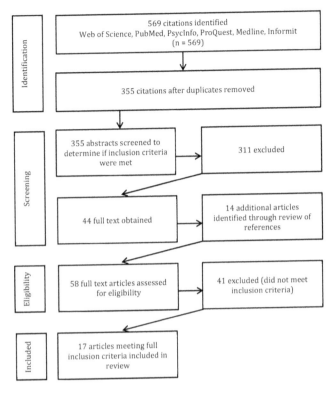

Figure 1. Literature review flowchart.

Overview of the studies

The majority of the studies focused on the impact on the individual who sustained the violence-related TBI ($n = 15$), with only two studies documenting impacts on family members (Arango-Lasprilla et al., 2008; Kreutzer, Marwitz, Hsu, Williams, & Riddick, 2007). Of the 17 articles, 12 were from the United States, published between 1998 and 2008, and using a mix of prospective and retrospective designs. There were four Canadian studies, all published between 2010 and 2013, three of which were retrospective, retrieving data from databases, medical records, and registry information. The one study from the United Kingdom, published in 1998, used prospective data.

The majority of studies were conducted among cohorts who had received inpatient rehabilitation (8 of 17 studies). Most of these studies were multi-center, drawing on units that were part of the TBI model systems (Dijkers, Harrison-Felix, & Marwitz, 2010). The next largest group was studies based in acute-care settings, ranging from single-center (e.g., Wagner et al., 2000) to population-based studies based on trauma registries (Kim et al., 2011). The other studies included two that recruited samples from single-center outpatient rehabilitation clinics and one that involved secondary analysis of data collected from three intervention trials.

The prevalence of violence-related TBIs, as a subset of all TBIs, varied between 6% and 26% within the studies (see Table 2). In examining these studies, the breakdown of violent versus nonviolent etiologies across these studies (see Table 2, column 6) does not typically add up to the total study samples (see Table 2, column 5), because some sample participants have not been included in these analyses (e.g., people with other forms of nontraumatic brain injury). The definitions of violence ranged from single-term global descriptors (e.g., violence, assault, gunshot) through to studies that used specific ICD–9CM E-codes (see Table 2). There was a national difference in the use of terminology, with the Canadian studies employing the terms *intentional* versus *nonintentional* violence (as reflected in the WHO definition), whereas the terminology within the U.S. studies generally did not include the dimension of intentionality.

Several other differences were noticeable in the approaches to definition across the studies that are likely to create unwanted variability in the prevalence reports. Many studies conflated self-inflicted and other-inflicted injuries, although the two types of behavior are quite different in the underlying motivation and circumstances. This concern is reflected in a minority of studies that did exclude self-inflicted injuries (e.g., Esselman et al., 2004; Kim et al., 2011; Schopp et al., 2006). All gunshot-related injuries were assumed to be violence-related (other-inflicted and self-inflicted) with the exception of one study that distinguished between intentional and accidental gunshot (Schopp et al., 2006). Similarly, falls were generally treated as a discrete nonviolent injury etiology with the exception of one study that recognized that some violence-related TBIs arise from pushing someone over (Bushnik, Hanks, Kreutzer, & Rosenthal, 2003).

The sample size across the studies was generally large in the context of rehabilitation studies. Most reports had samples ranging from greater than 100 through to 15,000 in the largest study. Almost all the studies focused on the acute phase or inpatient rehabilitation across the first year postinjury.

Five studies provided a breakdown of the different types of violence that led to the TBI. Two provided a simple breakdown of other-inflicted versus self-inflicted violence (Kim et al., 2011; Machamer et al., 2003). The other three provided more detailed breakdowns of the various types of assault (Gerhart et al., 2003; Harrison-Felix et al., 1998; Wagner et al., 2000) but there was little consensus across the findings (see Table 2).

Two studies (Bogner, Corrigan, Mysiw, Clinchot, & Fugate, 2001; Machamer et al., 2003) found that people with violence-related TBIs had significantly higher dropout rates, suggesting that this group might have been underrepresented in both studies. However, Machamer et al. (2003) conducted a multivariate analysis testing the strength of a range of demographic and psychosocial variables in predicting the likelihood of not being included in the study. Sex, age, and race were all significant individual predictors in the model, but violent etiology was not a significant predictor of study adherence.

Table 2. Studies examining violence-related traumatic brain injury.

Study	Study design	Service setting and source of data	Definition of violence	N, time since injury	Etiology and breakdown1
Arango-Lasprilla et al. (2008), U.S.	Retrospective longitudinal, multicenter	16 Traumatic Brain Injury Model Systems units (TBIMS; acute care through to inpatient [IP] rehabilitation); TBIMS national database	Gunshot, blunt assaults, other violence	977 (n = 969 where cause of injury known); 2 years	Violent (n = 31, 3%) Nonviolent (n = 714)
Bogner et al. (2001), U.S.	Retrospective longitudinal, single-center	TBI acute IP rehabilitation unit; Patient medical records and telephone surveys	Injury resulting from an assault or a gunshot wound, including unintentional gunshot wounds	351; 1 year	Violent (n = 53, 15%) Nonviolent (n = 298)
Bushnik et al. (2003), U.S.	Prospective longitudinal, multicenter	17 TBIMS units (acute care and IP rehabilitation); TBIMS national database	Not defined	1,170; 1 year	Violence (n = 250, 21%) Nonviolent (vehicle n = 629; falls n = 188; other n = 107)
Dagher et al. (2010), Canada	Retrospective cross-section single center	TBI Programme of the Montreal General Hospital (tertiary care center); Patient medical records	Assault cases excluded if mechanism of injury not clearly specified	415; Acute care phase	Assault (n = 91, 22%) Motor vehicle collision (MVC, n = 324)
Esselman et al. (2004), U.S.	Cross-section single center	Level 1 trauma center; Harborview Medical Center Trauma Registry	Not defined Based on ICD E-codes (not reported) Self-inflicted injury excluded	1,807; Acute care phase	Violent (n = 286, 16%) Nonviolent (n = 1,521)
Gerhart et al. (2003), U.S.	Retrospective longitudinal	Colorado hospitals Colorado Traumatic Brain Injury Registry and Follow-up System; Follow-up interviews	Interpersonal or self-inflicted violence including gunshot wounds, attacks with other objects, fights and altercations, and the intentional pushing of one person by another	1,802; 1 year	Violent (n = 112, 6%) Nonviolent (n = 1,689) Mechanisms for violent injuries (n = 112): 91.1% inflicted by others during assaults, attacks, or other acts of aggression (5% firearms; 48% knives, other sharp or cutting instruments, or

(Continued)

Table 2. Continued.

Study	Study design	Service setting and source of data	Definition of violence	N, time since injury	Etiology and breakdown[1]
					blunt objects; 47% assaults or pushes from high places); 7.9% self-inflicted (all gunshot wounds); 1.0% unknown
Hanks et al. (2003), U.S.	Prospective longitudinal	Acute hospitalization and inpatient rehabilitation at four TBIMS Centers; Medical records	All actions, either by self or by others, that caused a TBI (e.g., assault with a blunt or penetrating object, gunshot wound)	1,229; 1 and 2 years	Violent (n = 325, 26%); Nonviolent (n = 904)
Hanlon et al. (1999), U.S.	Prospective longitudinal	Outpatient concussion clinic; Neuropsychological evaluation	Assault	100; 3–40 months	Motor vehicle collisions (61%), falls (11%), assaults (10%), falling object (10%), sport/recreation (5%), pedestrian (3%)
Harrison-Felix et al. (1998), U.S.	Prospective longitudinal	Four TBIMS Centers (acute care and IP rehabilitation); TBIMS database	All self-inflicted and other person-inflicted causes; intentional use of weapons, attacks using vehicles, sports equipment (e.g., baseball bats), and other items	803; 1 year	Violent (n = 234); Nonviolent (n = 569); Mechanisms for violent injuries (n = 234) were 56% blunt assaults (e.g., blunt object, unarmed fight, jump), 23% penetrating objects (e.g., firearm injuries), 21% unknown
Kim et al. (2011), Canada	Retrospective cohort	Acute care hospitals in Ontario; Ontario Trauma Registry's minimal data set	Intentional injury: self-inflicted, homicide or assault (ICD E-codes E950, E960, E969, E979)	15,684; Acute care phase	Intentional (n = 1,770, 11%); Unintentional (n = 13,914); Of intentional injuries, other inflicted, 62%; self-inflicted, 38%
Kim, Bayley, et al. (2013), Canada	Prospective cohort	Inpatient rehabilitation; Discharge Abstract Database National Rehabilitation Reporting System	Intentional injury: physical assault (self-inflicted not included)	1,564; Acute care and rehabilitation phase	Intentional (n = 163, 10%); Unintentional (n = 1,401)
Kim, Colantonio, Dawson, and Bayley (2013), Canada	Retrospective cohort	Inpatient rehabilitation; Discharge Abstract Database National Rehabilitation Reporting System	Intentional injury: homicide or assault (ICD E-codes E960, E969, E979; self-inflicted not included)	243; 3–6 months	Intentional (n = 24, 10%); Unintentional (n = 219)

Study	Design	Setting / Data source	Definition	Sample; Follow-up	Etiology breakdown
Kreutzer et al. (2007), U.S.	Prospective longitudinal	Outpatient rehabilitation clinic; Interviews, medical records, questionnaire (General Health and History Questionnaire)	Violence or assault	120; 30–69 months	Violent (11%) Nonviolent
Machamer et al. (2003), U.S.	Secondary data analysis	Three prospective longitudinal trials; Outpatient settings	Suicide attempts and assaults	752; 1 year	Violent ($n = 113$, 15%) Nonviolent ($n = 631$) Violent injuries: assault ($n = 101$) and suicide attempts ($n = 12$) Significantly higher dropout rate at 1 year: violent (31%) vs. nonviolent (21%, $p < .05$; Multivariate analysis found that it was other factors (sex, age, and race) that predicted dropout rather than violent etiology
Schopp et al. (2006), U.S.	Prospective longitudinal	2 IP rehabilitation facilities, one acute rehabilitation hospital, one long-term rehabilitation hospital	Definite assault-related injury (evidence of intention to inflict harm); Probable assault-related injury and self-inflicted injuries were excluded	45; 1 year	Violent ($n = 19$, 42%) Nonviolent ($n = 26$)
Wagner et al. (2000), U.S.	Prospective cross-section	Level 1 trauma center; Carolinas Medical Center Trauma Registry	Intentional injury defined by an ICD-9 E-codes ranging from E950–E976	2,637; Acute care setting	Intentional ($n = 469$, 17.8%) Unintentional ($n = 2,168$) Intentional etiologies ($n = 469$) included gunshot wounds (35%), assault (35%), stabbing (3%), other (explosive, jumping, suicide; 27%)
Wenden et al. (1998), UK	Prospective longitudinal	Hospital trauma service; Oxford Head Injury Service	Assault	625 ($n = 478$ at follow up); 6 months	Assault ($n = 90$, 14%) Nonassaults ($n = 417$)

Note: The breakdown of violent versus nonviolent etiologies (column 6) does not typically add up to the total sample (column 5), because some sample participants have not been included in these analyses (e.g., people with other forms of nontraumatic brain injury). ICD = International Classification of Diseases.

Demographic and psychosocial profile of violence-related TBI

The review found a number of premorbid and demographic features that were strongly associated with individuals who sustained a violence-related TBI (see Table 3). Of the 15 articles focusing on the individual, 10 specifically tested demographic details between violent and nonviolent TBI. Despite the high baseline of males compared to females after TBI (often at a ratio of 3 to 1), 8 of the 10 studies reported that a significantly higher proportion of males were represented among violent injuries compared to nonviolent injuries.

Next, the U.S.-based studies consistently found that the proportion of non-White or minority races was significantly higher compared to people of White racial background in the violence-related TBI group, although this finding was not observed in Canada (Dagher et al., 2010) or the United Kingdom. In the six studies that reported on age, there was no consistent pattern. Two studies found that people in adult age bands, 26 to 45 years old (Harrison-Felix et al., 1998) and 25 to 34 years old (Gerhart et al., 2003), had a higher risk of violence-related TBI compared to people of younger age (i.e., late adolescence and early adulthood). Three other studies (Dagher, Habra, Lamoureux, de Guise, & Feyz, 2010; Esselman et al., 2004; Hanks et al., 2003), though, found statistically significant between-group differences in mean ages (violence-related TBI younger than TBI from nonviolent causes), but as the mean differences only ranged from 1 to 7 years, these differences might not be clinically significant.

There was consistency in findings that people with violence-related TBIs were significantly more likely than the nonviolent group to be unemployed at the time of the injury. However, there was little conclusive evidence to date at $p < .01$ of differences in education levels between the two groups. Prior alcohol and prior drug abuse were significantly more common among violence-related TBIs in five studies, as were a preinjury history of arrests. Articles reporting on marital status or the proportions of people living alone postinjury suggest that significantly more individuals who sustained violence-related TBIs were single or living alone. Finally, one study also found that people with violence-related TBIs were significantly more likely to have been the victim of violence prior to the TBI (Schopp et al., 2006).

Injury and injury-related factors

The three variables examined in this category were injury severity, blood alcohol levels at admission to the hospital, and the presence of other traumatic injuries (apart from the TBI). Nine of the 15 studies that focused on individuals investigated one or more of these variables. Starting with injury severity, the three strongest severity classification measures are the Glasgow Coma Scale (GCS; Teasdale & Jennett, 1976), duration of loss of consciousness

Table 3. Premorbid and demographic features (all findings at $p < .01$ or Bonferroni corrected).

Study	Sex, % male V vs. NV	Race, non-White V vs. NV	Age (years) V vs. NV	Not married V vs. NV	Unemployed at injury V vs. NV	Education V vs. NV	Prior alcohol abuse V vs. NV	Prior drug abuse V vs. NV	Other V vs. NV
Harrison-Felix et al. (1998)	86% vs. 74%	71% vs. 42%	26–45; 57% vs. 41%	91% vs. 69%	50% vs. 24%	ns trend	NR	NR	Live alone 29% vs. 16%
Bogner et al. (2001)	96% vs. 76%	32% vs. 4%	ns	ns	51% vs. 20%	ns trend	ns trend	NR	NR
Hanks et al. (2003)	86% vs. 72%	74% vs. 46%	37 ± 17 vs. 36 ± 13	NR	44% vs. 21%	<high school degree 48% vs. 39%	NR	NR	NR
Gerhart et al. (2003)	83% vs. 67%	40% vs. 14%	25–34; 26% vs. 18%	84% vs. 64%	ns	NR	28% vs. 11%	ns	Previous TBI ns
Bushnik et al. (2003)	ns	56% vs. NV	ns	86% vs. NV	42% vs. NV	ns	ns	46% vs. NV	History of arrest 60% vs. NV
Machamer et al. (2003)	89% vs. 77%	37% vs. 12%	ns	ns	NR	ns	40% vs. 23%	ns	Preexisting conditions, yes 80% vs. 61%; History of arrest, yes 67% vs. 40%
Esselman et al. (2004)	91% vs. 62%	44% vs. 20%	34.8.0 ± 11.5 vs. 39.5 ± 18.4	NR	NR	NR	NR	NR	NR
Schopp et al. (2006)	ns	37% vs. 0%	ns	ns	53% vs. 8%	ns	ns	78% vs. 38%	Perpetrator violence, 57% vs. 16%; Victim of violence, 89% vs. 21%
Dagher et al. (2010)	92% vs. 67%	ns	35.0 ± 13.3 vs. 42.0 ± 19.6	ns trend	ns trend	ns at .01	54% vs. 21%	43% vs. 20%	Prior criminal record ns
Kim, Bayley, et al. (2013)	92% vs. 75%	NR	16–24, 32% vs. 29%	NR	56% vs. 35%	NR	NR	NR	Live alone, 28% vs. 17%

Note: V = violent; NV = nonviolent; ns = nonsignificant; NR = not reported; TBI = traumatic brain injury.

(LOC), and duration of posttraumatic amnesia (PTA), with the latter two measured in days (Teasdale, 1995). These measures are routinely assessed in inpatient rehabilitation and outpatient settings.

The studies that examined injury severity (GCS, LOC, PTA) found no significant differences in injury severity between violence- and non-violence-related etiologies of TBI (see Table 4). In the absence of these frontline measures, studies in acute settings fall back on the degree of injury to the head region as measured by the Abbreviated Injury Scale, or length of stay in hospital as proxies for injury severity, but these two approaches are far from ideal. Studies that relied on these measures were not considered for the injury severity variable in this review.

In contrast to injury severity, there were consistent findings that people admitted with violence-related TBIs had significantly higher blood alcohol levels than people with nonviolent etiologies. These differences were clinically important in one study that found significantly greater proportions of people had blood alcohol levels above the legal limit as defined within their specific jurisdiction (Esselman et al., 2004). Finally, two studies found that people with

Table 4. Injury and injury-related factors (all findings at $p < .01$ or Bonferroni corrected).

Study	Injury severity V vs. NV	BAL at admission V vs. NV	Other traumatic injuries V vs. NV
Harrison-Felix et al. (1998)	GCS at ED admission, 9.6 vs. 8.3 Highest GCS in first 24 hr, 10.9 vs. 9.7	V vs. NV, ns	NR
Hanks et al. (2003)	Ns	93 mg/dL vs. 67.1 mg/dL	NR
Gerhart et al. (2003)	GCS scores, ns	NR	NR
Bushnik et al. (2003)	GCS at ED admission and highest GCS in first 24 hr V > vehicle, loss of consciousness, duration of posttraumatic amnesia, ns	NR	NR
Machamer et al. (2003)	GCS, ns	142 mg/dL vs. 87 mg/dL	NR
Esselman et al. (2004)	GCS, ns	(≥80 mg/dL) legal limit, 40% vs. 25%	Highest other (nonhead) body system, AIS ≥ 3, 18% v. 39%; AIS level 4 (head), 47% vs. 34%
Schopp et al. (2006)	Loss of consciousness, ns	NR	NR
Dagher et al. (2010)	ns	33.5 ± 28.7 mg/dL vs. 10.9 ± 21.4 mg/dL	Polytrauma, 37.5% vs. 84.5%; ISS, 23.3 ± 12.2 vs. 33.1 ± 12.1
Kim, Bayley, et al. (2013)	NR	NR	Number of comorbidities, ns

Note: V = violent; NV = nonviolent; GCS = Glasgow Coma Scale; ns = nonsignificant; NR = not recorded; ED = Emergency Department; BAL = blood alcohol level; AIS = Abbreviated Injury Scale; ISS = Injury Severity Score; mg/dL = milligram per deciliter.

nonviolent TBIs had significantly higher rates of trauma to other body systems as measured by the Abbreviated Injury Scale and Injury Severity Score.

Outcomes from violence-related TBIs

Outcomes were reported in 11 of 15 studies (see Table 5). The types of variables included the presence of neurological symptoms (e.g., dizziness, headaches), neuropsychological impairments (e.g., attention, memory, executive functions), and current employment status. Validated measures were also employed to assess functional status or levels of community participation, most commonly at one or more of three set time points (admission to inpatient rehabilitation, discharge from inpatient rehabilitation, some subsequent follow-up time point). Finally, some attempts were made to capture more global aspects of individuals' overall functioning.

Two studies investigated the presence of ongoing symptoms, with one finding people with violence-related TBIs were more likely to report changes to vision and taste at 1 year postinjury (Gerhart et al., 2003) and have significantly higher overall symptom scores on the Rivermead Post-Concussional Questionnaire (Wenden et al., 1998). Three studies examined the presence of neuropsychological impairments but in most cases the comparisons were nonsignificant across tests of intelligence, memory, premorbid reading ability (a commonly used proxy for levels of premorbid intelligence) and executive function, with the exception of one finding in the study by Hanlon et al. (1999) that people with violence-related TBI performed more poorly on the Trail Making Test B, a measure of executive function.

Five studies reported on postinjury employment status, and although two smaller studies found significantly higher levels of unemployment among the violence-related TBIs (Bushnik et al., 2003; Schopp et al., 2006), this was not found at the $p < .01$ level in the three larger studies (Gerhart et al., 2003; Harrison-Felix et al., 1998; Machamer et al., 2003). One study (Dagher et al., 2010) reported outcome status at discharge from acute care for a group that mostly did not go onto inpatient or outpatient rehabilitation. People with violence-related TBIs had significantly better outcomes at discharge on the Glasgow Outcome Scale–Extended compared to the nonviolence group, with the mean score (3.57) sitting just over the moderate disability range.

The only measure reported at admission to inpatient rehabilitation was the Functional Independence Measure (FIM; Linacre, Heinemann, Wright, Granger, & Hamilton, 1994). The FIM is a measure that rates the ability of a person to independently perform his or her own self-care, bowel and bladder function, personal mobility, cognition and communication, and appropriate social interactions within a social setting. Higher scores indicate greater independence, with the total score ranging from 18 to 126, with two subscales: FIM Motor (13 items, 13–91) and FIM Cognition (5 items,

Table 5. Outcomes (all findings at $p < .01$ or Bonferroni corrected).

Study	Symptoms V vs. NV	NP impair-ments V vs. NV	Current un-employment V vs. NV	Measures at acute care discharge V vs. NV	Measures at IP rehab admission V vs. NV	Measures at IP rehab discharge V vs. NV	Measures at follow-up V vs. NV	Behavior/overall function V vs. NV
Harrison-Felix et al. (1998)	NR	NR	ns	NR	FIM Motor, 46 vs. 40	FIM, ns	1-year follow-up FIM, ns; CIQ Social subscale, 6.8 vs. 8.0; Productivity, 2.3 vs 3.2; Total, 13.3 vs. 16.0	Living alone/not with family, 45% vs. 32%
Wenden et al. (1998)	Rivermead Post-Concussion Questionnaire, 13.7 ± 13.9 vs. 6.3 ± 9.6	NR	NR	NR	NR	NR	NR	Rivermead Head Injury Follow-up Questionnaire, 7.0 ± 8.4 vs. 3.0 ± 5.6
Hanlon et al. (1999)	NR	Executive function Trail Making B, V < NV	NR	NR	NR	NR	NR	NR
Wagner et al. (2000)	NR	NR	NR	NR	NR	NR	1-year follow-up CIQ Total score V < NV	NR
Gerhart et al. (2003)	1-year follow-up, Vision, 47% vs. 25%; Taste, 26% vs. 16%	NR	ns	NR	NR	NR	1-year follow-up CHART Social integration, 80.3 vs. 86.4; Economic self-sufficiency, 70.1 vs. 83.3; Total, 501.8 vs. 531.4	NR
Bushnik et al. (2003)	NR	NR	70% vs. NV	NR	NR	DRS, FIM, ns	1-year follow-up DRS, 3.8 ± 4.1 vs. 2.4 ± 3.1; CIQ Total, 12.9 ± 6.2 vs. 16.1 ± 5.8	FIM total change (Admission–discharge), 38.6 ± 19.5 vs. 44.2 ± 22.2;

Study							
Machamer et al. (2003)	NR	Verbal intelligence; Performance intelligence; Trails A and B; Stroop A and B; Recall, all ns	ns	NR	NR	NR	Total change: discharge –1 year postinjury DRS, 2.3 ± 3.3 vs. 3.4 ± 3.0; FIM total, 15.4 ± 15.5 vs. 19.6 ± 17.3 Sickness Impact Score, ns Brief Symptom Inventory Trend at p < .5
Schopp et al. (2006)	NR	WAIS–R–7[a] WRAT3 WMS–R RAVLT Trails A, B, all ns	ns Access Supplemental Security Income 61% vs. 12%	NR	FIM, ns	FIM, ns	1-year follow-up Access psychiatric treatment, ns; Legal history, ns
Dagher et al. (2010)	NR	NR	NR	Glasgow Outcome Scale–Extended, 3.57 vs. 4.29; FIM, ns NR	NR	NR	NR
Kim, Bayley, et al. (2013)	NR	NR	NR	NR	FIM total, 88.9 ± 27.2 vs. 79.6 ± 30.2; FIM Motor, 68.1 ± 22.3 vs. 59.5 ± 25.0	FIM total, ns at <.01; FIM Motor, 84.9 (12.8) vs. 80.5 (17.3)	FIM total change (Admission – discharge) 22.4 ± 21.1 vs. 27.3 ± 23.2

(Continued)

Table 5. Continued.

Study	Symptoms V vs. NV	NP impair-ments V vs. NV	Current un-employment V vs. NV	Measures at acute care discharge V vs. NV	Measures at IP rehab admission V vs. NV	Measures at IP rehab discharge V vs. NV	Measures at follow-up V vs. NV	Behavior/overall function V vs. NV
Kim, Colantonio, et al. (2013)	NR	NR	NR	NR	NR	NR	3–6 month follow-up RNLI Total score, V < NV; Daily functioning subscale, V < NV; Recreation, V < NV; Family role, V < NV	NR

Note: V = violence; NV = nonviolence; NR = not reported; *ns* = nonsignificant; CHART = Craig Handicap Assessment and Reporting Technique; FIM = Functional Independence Measure; CIQ = Community Integration Questionnaire; DRS = Disability Rating Scale; WAIS–R–7 = Wechsler Adult Intelligence Scale–Revised–7; WRAT3 = Wide Range Achievement Test–3; WMS–R = Wechsler Memory Scale–Revised; RAVLT = Rey Auditory Verbal Learning Test; RNLI = Reintegration to Normal Living Index; IP = inpatient; NP = neuropsychologist.
*a*Trend = *p* < .05.

5–35). Three studies reported admission FIM (Harrison-Felix et al., 1998; Kim, Bayley, Dawson, Mollayeva, & Colantonio, 2013; Schopp et al., 2006), with two finding that people with violence-related TBIs were significantly more independent than people with nonviolent TBIs (Harrison-Felix et al., 1998; Kim et al., 2013). One study also found the violence group had higher FIM total scores (Kim et al., 2013). There were no significant differences in FIM Cognition scores. At the point of discharge from inpatient rehabilitation, most of these differences had disappeared, with only one study finding a significant difference in the FIM Motor scores (Kim et al., 2013), with the violence-related TBI group being more independent. Finally, people with non-violence-related TBIs made significantly greater gains in functional status (FIM scores) between admission and discharge.

At the follow-up time point, people with violence-related TBI demonstrated significantly poorer scores in scales evaluating productivity, economic self-sufficiency, social integration, and recreation (Bushnik et al., 2003; Harrison-Felix et al., 1998; Wagner et al., 2000). These results were found across a range of measures of participation (see Table 5). Follow-up was commonly conducted at 1 year postinjury.

Service pathways and financial costs

The final domain examined for individuals with violence-related TBIs were the service pathways and financial costs (reported in 8 of 15 studies). Variables reported included acute length of stay, discharge disposition from the acute hospital setting, length of stay in inpatient rehabilitation, service-related costs, payer status, and other heterogeneous variables (see Table 6). People with violence-related TBIs had significantly shorter lengths of stay in both acute (Esselman et al., 2004; Kim et al., 2013) and inpatient rehabilitation settings (Harrison-Felix et al., 1998). They were also more likely to be discharged home instead of referred to rehabilitation (Dagher et al., 2010; Esselman et al., 2004). Four studies reported that violence-related injury treatment was more likely to be funded from the public purse than from private insurance (Esselman et al., 2004; Gerhart et al., 2003; Harrison-Felix et al., 1998; Schopp et al., 2006). Kim et al. (2011) found that individuals with intentional injuries had higher rates of discharge against medical advice and they associated this with a younger population who had a premorbid history of alcohol and drug abuse.

Impact on families or informal caregivers

Two studies were identified that reported on the impact of violence-related TBI on postinjury marital stability (Arango-Lasprilla et al., 2008; Kreutzer et al., 2007). In a multivariate model, Arango-Lasprilla et al. (2008) found that over the first 2 years postinjury, people with violence-related TBI were three

Table 6. Costs (all findings at $p < .01$ or Bonferroni corrected).

Study	Acute length of stay (days) V vs. NV	Discharge disposition: Referral to IP rehabilitation? V vs. NV	IP rehab length of stay (days) V vs. NV	Costs V vs. NV	Payer status V vs. NV	Other V vs. NV
Harrison-Felix et al. (1998)	20 vs. 25	NR	33 vs. 41	1996 USD acute length of stay, $81,000 vs. $112,000	Medicaid acute hospital, >50% vs. 21%; Medicaid IP rehab, >50% vs. 21%	NR
Gerhart et al. (2003)	NR	Discharge disposition, ns	NR	NR	Government health care funding, ns	V vs. NV Rehabilitation/ therapy service use, ns
Bushnik et al. (2003)	ns	NR	ns	NR	NR	NR
Esselman et al. (2004)	5.5 ± 6.7 vs. 9.2 ± 10.6	Rehab vs. home odds ratio = 0.54	NR	NR	Medicaid acute hospital, 54% vs. 28%	NR
Schopp et al. (2006)	NR	NR	NR	NR	Medicaid rehab, 89% vs. 33%	NR
Dagher et al. (2010)	ns	Discharged home, 28.9% vs. 11.5%	NR	NR	NR	V vs. NV Orthopedic surgery, 4.4% vs. 34.6%
Kim et al. (2011)	NR	NR	NR	NR	NR	DAMA vs. regular discharge: other-inflicted, 18% vs, 7%; self-inflicted, 8% vs. 4%
Kim, Bayley, et al. (2013)	48.4 ± 86.6 vs. 56.8 ± 100.6	NR	ns	NR	NR	Home without services, 59% vs. 52%

Note: V = violent; NV = vonviolent; IP = inpatient; USD = U.S. dollars; NR = not reported; ns = nonsignificant; DAMA = discharge against medical advice.

times more likely to experience marital breakdown compared to people with nonviolent TBI (odds ratio = 2.99, 95% CI [1.55, 5.75]). Similarly, Kreutzer et al. (2007) found that people with violence-related TBI were three times more likely to have experienced marital breakdown up to 8 years post-TBI (still married, 7 violent versus 93 nonviolent; separated or divorced, 24 violent versus 76 nonviolent; statistically significant, chi-square).

Discussion

Across acute and rehabilitation service settings, the prevalence of violence-related TBI ranged between 3% and 26% as a proportion of all causes of TBI. There was a consistent profile of people at greatest risk of sustaining violence-related TBI and the associated outcomes. People sustaining TBIs through violence were more likely to be male, be unemployed at the time of injury, have a preinjury history of substance abuse and prior arrests, and to be single or living alone. In the context of the United States, people at risk were also more likely to be from non-White or minority racial groups, but this finding did not generalize to other countries. The violence-etiology group was also more likely to have elevated blood alcohol levels on admission to the hospital, but less non-head-related polytrauma compared to people sustaining TBI by other etiologies. There were few differences in outcomes based on symptom reports, neuropsychological tests, or functional measures. However, the violence-related TBI group generally reported poorer FIM gain during inpatient rehabilitation than nonviolent groups, and lower scores in the domain of participation at 1 year follow-up, particularly in areas of productivity and social integration. In terms of navigating systems, people with violence-related TBI were more likely to draw on government-related supports (Medicaid) than private insurance and were more likely to be discharged home. Finally, the marriages of people with violence-related TBIs were at greater risk of breaking down postinjury compared to those of people with TBI from other etiologies.

Overall, the prevalence data might be either overestimates (due to some studies aggregating self-inflicted violence with other-inflicted violence; aggregating intentional with accidental gunshot) or underestimates (e.g., some studies not taking into account that falls could also be due to violence) of the true rate of violence-related TBI. This problem was reflected particularly in decisions about which ICD E-codes (external causes of injury) would be included as representing violence (e.g., see Bushnik et al., 2003; Esselman et al., 2004; Harrison-Felix et al., 1998). Further investigation as to whether self-inflicted and other-inflicted etiologies have sufficient commonality to be grouped together will help improve consistency for future investigations into the prevalence of violence-related TBI.

It was clear from the premorbid and demographic data that violence-related TBI was strongly associated with a particular socioeconomic profile

(Bogner et al., 2001; Hanks et al., 2003; Harrison-Felix et al., 1998; Kim et al., 2013). However, the evidence for some variables (e.g., a younger age group, poorer education levels) was not as strong once the more stringent criterion of $p < .01$ was applied, compared to variables such as sex, race, and preinjury employment status. The findings support the notion that people among poorer socioeconomic groups might be at greater risk of sustaining violent TBI (Harrison-Felix et al., 1998).

This socioeconomic profile provides a confounding factor in determining the impact of violence-related TBI on outcomes including participation in health services and 1 year functional and participation status. Multivariate analyses in some studies (Bogner et al., 2001; Gerhart et al., 2003; Harrison-Felix et al., 1998) found that socioeconomic characteristics were significant predictors for service use or scores on participation scales, rather than the injury etiology per se. Higher dropout rates were also noted in some research studies among participants with violence-related TBI compared to people sustaining their TBI through other etiologies (Bogner et al., 2001; Machamer et al., 2003). This raises the concern that the samples in the studies identified in this review might not be representative of all people who sustain violence-related TBIs.

Premorbid alcohol abuse is associated with TBI more generally (Corrigan, 1995, cited in Bogner et al., 2001). The studies in this review have extended this, finding a specific association between alcohol abuse and violence-related TBI, consistent with research in the general community of the links between alcohol and violence (Homel, Carvolth, Hauritz, McIlwain, & Teague, 2004). The frequent presence of elevated blood alcohol levels at the time of injury is also well established in the TBI field (Corrigan, 1995, cited in Bogner et al., 2001), but the significantly higher levels associated with violence-related TBIs compared to other TBI etiologies have not been widely reported.

The review did not find a consistent difference in the pattern of injury severity, despite suggestions that people with violence-related TBIs might report less severe injuries. For example Alexander (1995, cited in Hanlon et al., 1999) suggested that the inertial force generated by a blow to a stationary head is not equivalent to the inertial force generated by instantaneous deceleration typically experienced in road crashes. However, the findings from most studies that reported on this issue were inconclusive. This might be due in part to few studies being able to employ the best indicators of initial injury severity (duration of PTA, LOC, or both) and therefore further research is required. There has also been discussion of whether people surviving violence-related TBIs due to penetrating injuries (e.g., gunshot wounds) might have less severe injuries than people experiencing blunt-force trauma (e.g., punch to the head), but one of the few studies to investigate this found little difference in outcomes between the two subgroups (Zafonte et al., 1997). The higher level of polytrauma observed among people sustaining nonviolent types of TBI (e.g., road-related) has also been observed in other studies (Grosswasser et al.,

1990, cited in Esselman et al., 2004), and is supported by the much higher rates of acute orthopedic surgery reported by this group (Dagher et al., 2010). These findings are consistent with the stronger forces associated with road crashes.

The overall lack of difference between violence- and non-violence-related TBIs across most domains of outcomes reported in the studies is consistent with the lack of difference in initial injury severity. The significant differences in the amount of FIM gain observed during the episode of inpatient rehabilitation might reflect the lower levels of polytrauma experienced after violence-related TBIs. One domain rarely investigated among outcomes were the emotional consequences (with the exception of Machamer et al., 2003), and it could be that people who sustain the TBI through violence might experience greater levels of posttraumatic stress or other emotional sequelae associated with exposure to violence. Finally, the majority of studies only reported on outcomes up to the end of the first year postinjury, so little is known about possible longer term consequences.

People with violence-related TBI generally had a shorter length of stay when admitted to acute care or inpatient rehabilitation (Esselman et al., 2004; Harrison-Felix et al., 1998; Kim et al., 2013). In the United States, there was strong evidence that people with violence-related TBIs were more likely to draw on Medicaid funding (Esselman et al., 2004; Harrison-Felix et al., 1998; Schopp et al., 2006). This is consistent with the demographic features reported previously that suggest a lower socioeconomic status.

The review found no studies that specifically investigated the impact of violence-related TBI on family members or informal caregivers, a paucity of research also observed by Arango-Lasprilla et al. (2008). However, the two identified studies both found that violence-related TBI had an independent impact on postinjury marital stability. Neither study was able to suggest a reason for this, apart from the broader impact of associated difficulties in productivity reported by people with violence-related TBI (Kreutzer et al., 2007). The results from the studies are consistent with one of the reports that focused on the individual with TBI (Bushnik et al., 2003).

In terms of the practice-based implications, studies within the review suggested that people with violence-related TBI comprised a distinct clinical subgroup within TBI (Kim et al., 2013). Particular approaches to improving the quality of life for this group need to be a focus for service providers (Hanks et al., 2003). To date, no specialized interventions have been reported (Kim et al., 2013) and this is an important area for future research.

References

Anderson, M. I., Simpson, G. K., & Morey, P. J. (2013). The impact of neurobehavioral impairment on family functioning and the psychological well-being of male versus female caregivers of relatives with severe traumatic brain injury: Multi-group analysis. *Journal of Head Trauma Rehabilitation, 28,* 453–463. doi:10.1097/htr.0b013e31825d6087

Arango-Lasprilla, J. C., Ketchum, J. M., Dezfulian, T., Kreutzer, J. S., O'Neil-Pirozzi, T. M., Hammond, F., & Jha, A. (2008). Predictors of marital stability 2 years following traumatic brain injury. *Brain Injury, 22,* 565–574. doi:10.1080/02699050802172004

Arksey, H., & O'Malley, L. (2005). Scoping studies: Towards a methodological framework. *International Journal of Social Research Methodology, 8*(1), 19–32. doi:10.1080/1364557032000119616

Atkinson, B. (2014, September 4). Australians falling victim to random violent assaults in public. Retrieved from http://www.news.com.au/national/australians-falling-victim-to-random-violent-assaults-in-public/news-story/06f49b7d0dbfaaa892b95df2a87dcdf8

Berg, C. (2014, August 19). Mandatory sentencing: A king hit for courts. Retrieved from http://www.abc.net.au/news/2014-08-19/berg-mandatory-sentencing-a-king-hit-for-courts/5681594

Bogner, J. A., Corrigan, J. D., Mysiw, W. J., Clinchot, D., & Fugate, L. (2001). A comparison of substance abuse and violence in the prediction of long-term rehabilitation outcomes after traumatic brain injury. *Archives of Physical Medicine and Rehabilitation, 82,* 571–577. doi:10.1053/apmr.2001.22340

Boycott, N., Yeoman, P., & Vesey, P. (2013). Factors associated with strain in carers of people with traumatic brain injury. *Journal of Head Trauma Rehabilitation, 28,* 106–115. doi:10.1097/HTR.0b013e31823fe07e

Burke, H., Degeneffe, C. E., & Olney, M. F. (2009). A new disability for rehabilitation counselors: Iraq war veterans with traumatic brain injury and post-traumatic stress disorder. *The Journal of Rehabilitation, 75*(3), 5–14.

Bushnik, T., Hanks, R. A., Kreutzer, J., & Rosenthal, M. (2003). Etiology of traumatic brain injury: Characterization of differential outcomes up to 1 year postinjury. *Archives of Physical Medicine and Rehabilitation, 84*, 255–262. doi:10.1053/apmr.2003.50092

Caro, D. H. J. (2011). Traumatic brain injury care systems: 2020 transformational challenges. *Global Journal of Health Science, 3*(1), 19–29. doi:10.5539/gjhs.v3n1p19

Carter, R. E., Lubinsky, J., & Domholdt, E. (2011). *Rehabilitation research,* (4th ed.). St. Louis, MO: Elsevier Sanders.

Colantonio, A., Saverino, C., Zagorski, B., Swaine, B., Lewko, J., Jaglal, S., & Vernich, L. (2010). Hospitalizations and emergency department visits for TBI in Ontario. *The Canadian Journal of Neurological Sciences, 37*, 783–790.

Dagher, J. H., Habra, N., Lamoureux, J., de Guise, E., & Feyz, M. (2010). Global outcome in acute phase of treatment following moderate-to-severe traumatic brain injury from motor vehicle collisions vs assaults. *Brain Injury, 24*, 1389–1398. doi:10.3109/02699052.2010.523042

Degeneffe, C. E. (2001). Family caregiving and traumatic brain injury. *Health and Social Work, 26*, 257–268. doi:10.1093/hsw/26.4.257

Dijkers, M. P., Harrison-Felix, C., & Marwitz, J. H. (2010). The traumatic brain injury model systems: History and contributions to clinical service and research. *Journal of Head Trauma Rehabilitation, 25*, 81–91. doi:10.1097/htr.0b013e3181cd3528

Dow, A. (2013, December 2). King-hit deaths prompt new law push. *The Age.* Retrieved from http://www.theage.com.au/victoria/kinghit-deaths-prompt-new-law-push-20131201-2yjv0.html

Elbaum, J. (2007). Acquired brain injury and the family. In J. Elbaum, & D. Benson (Eds.), *Acquired brain injury,* (pp. 275–285). New York, NY: Springer.

Esselman, P. C., Dikmen, S. S., Bell, K., & Temkin, N. R. (2004). Access to inpatient rehabilitation after violence-related traumatic brain injury. *Archives of Physical Medicine and Rehabilitation, 85*, 1445–1449. doi:10.1016/j.apmr.2003.10.018

Farrow, L. (2015, June 12). NSW man sentenced over one-punch kill. *The Australian.* Retrieved from http://www.theaustralian.com.au/news/latest-news/nsw-man-sentenced-over-one-punch-kill/story-fn3dxiwe-1227395135712

Faul, M., Xu, L., Wald, M. M., & Coronado, V. (2010). *Traumatic brain injury in the United States: Emergency department visits, hospitalization and death 2002–2006.* Atlanta, GA: Centers for Disease Control and Prevention. Retrieved from http://www.cdc.gov/traumaticbraininjury/pdf/blue_book.pdf

Federal Bureau of Investigation. (2014). *2014 crime in the United States.* Retrieved from https://www.fbi.gov/news/stories/2015/september/latest-crime-stats-released/latest-crime-states-released

Finkelstein, E. A., Corso, P. S., & Miller, T. R. (2006). *The incidence and economic burden of injuries in the United States.* Oxford, UK: Oxford University Press.

Freedy, J. R., Resnick, H. S., Kilpatrick, D. G., Danksy, B. S., & Tidwell, R. P. (1994). The psychological adjustment of recent crime victims in the criminal justice system. *Journal of Interpersonal Violence, 9*, 450–468. doi:10.1177/088626094009004002

Gerhart, K. A., Mellick, D. C., & Weintraub, A. H. (2003). Violence-related traumatic brain injury: A population-based study. *The Journal of Trauma: Injury, Infection, and Critical Care, 55*, 1045–1053. doi:10.1097/01.TA.0000044353.69681.96

Hall, K. M., Karzmark, P., Stevens, M., Englander, J., O'Hare, P., & Wright, J. (1994). Family stressors in traumatic brain injury: A two-year follow-up. *Archives of Physical Medicine and Rehabilitation, 75*, 876–884. doi:10.1016/0003-9993(94)90112-0

Hanks, R. A., Wood, D. L., Millis, S., Harrison-Felix, C., Pierce, C. A., Rosenthal, M., … Kreutzer, J. (2003). Violent traumatic brain injury: Occurrence, patient characteristics, and risk factors from the traumatic brain injury model systems project. *Archives of Physical Medicine and Rehabilitation, 84*, 249–254. doi:10.1053/apmr.2003.50096

Hanlon, R. E., Demery, J. A., Martinovich, Z., & Kelly, J. P. (1999). Effects of acute injury characteristics on neuropsychological status and vocational outcome following mild traumatic brain injury. *Brain Injury, 13*, 873–887. doi:10.1080/026990599121070

Harrison-Felix, C., Zafonte, R., Mann, N., Dijkers, M., Englander, J., & Kreutzer, J. (1998). Brain injury as a result of violence: Preliminary findings from the traumatic brain injury model systems. *Archives of Physical Medicine and Rehabilitation, 79*, 730–737. doi:10.1016/S0003-9993(98)90348-3

Helps, Y. L. M., Henley, G., & Harrison, J. E. (2008). *Hospital separations due to traumatic brain injury, Australia 2004–05.* Canberra, Australia: Australian Institute of Health and Welfare.

Homel, R., Carvolth, R., Hauritz, M., McIlwain, G., & Teague, R. (2004). Making licensed venues safer for patrons: What environmental factors should be the focus of interventions? *Drug and Alcohol Review, 23*, 19–29. doi:10.1080/09595230410001645529

Kim, H., Bayley, M., Dawson, D., Mollayeva, T., & Colantonio, A. (2013). Characteristics and functional outcomes of brain injury caused by physical assault in Canada: A population-based study from an inpatient rehabilitation setting. *Disability and Rehabilitation, 35*, 2213–2220. doi:10.3109/09638288.2013.774063

Kim, H., & Colantonio, A. (2008). Intentional traumatic brain injury in Ontario, Canada. *Journal of Trauma: Injury, Infection and Critical Care, 65*, 1287–1292. doi:10.1097/TA.0b013e31817196f5

Kim, H., Colantonio, A., Bayley, M., & Dawson, D. (2011). Discharge against medical advice after traumatic brain injury: Is intentional injury a predictor. *The Journal of Trauma: Injury, Infection, and Critical Care, 71*, 1219–1225. doi:10.1097/ta.0b013e3182190fa6

Kim, H., Colantonio, A., Dawson, D., & Bayley, M. (2013). Community integration outcomes after traumatic brain injury due to physical assault. *Canadian Journal of Occupational Therapy, 80*(1), 49–58.

Kreutzer, J. S., Marwitz, J. H., Hsu, N., Williams, K., & Riddick, A. (2007). Marital stability after brain injury: An investigation and analysis. *NeuroRehabilitation, 22*, 53–59.

Krug, E. G., Dahlberg, L. L., Mercy, J. A., Zwi, A. B., & Lozano, R. (2002). *World report on violence and health.* Geneva, Switzerland: World Health Organization. Retrieved from http://apps.who.int/iris/bitstream/10665/42495/1/9241545615_eng.pdf

Levac, D., Colquhoun, H., & O'Brien, K. K. (2010). Scoping studies: Advancing the methodology. *Implementation Science, 5*(69), 1–9. doi:10.1186/1748-5908-5-69

Linacre, J. M., Heinemann, A. W., Wright, B. D., Granger, C. V., & Hamilton, B. B. (1994). The structure and stability of the functional independence measure. *Archives of Physical Medicine and Rehabilitation, 75*, 127–132.

Linnarsson, J. R., Benzein, E., & Arestedt, K. (2014). Nurses' views of forensic care in emergency departments and their attitudes, and involvement of family members. *Journal of Clinical Nursing, 24*(1–2), 266–274. doi:10.1111/jocn.12638

Machamer, J. E., Temkin, N. R., & Dikmen, S. S. (2003). Neurobehavioral outcome in persons with violent or nonviolent traumatic brain injury. *Journal of Head Trauma Rehabilitation, 18*, 387–397. doi:10.1097/00001199-200309000-00001

Picenna, L., Pattuwage, L., Gruen, R., & Bragge, P. (2014). *Briefing document: Optimizing support for informal carers of the long-term disabled to enhance resilience and sustainability.* Retrieved from http://www.ntriforum.org.au

Ponsford, J., Olver, J., Ponsford, M., & Nelms, R. (2003). Long-term adjustment of families following traumatic brain injury where comprehensive rehabilitation has been provided. *Brain Injury, 17,* 453–468. doi:10.1080/0269905031000070143

Rosenberg, M. L., & Fenley, M. A. (Eds.). (1991). *Violence in America: A public health approach.* New York, NY: Oxford University Press.

Schopp, L. H., Good, G. E., Barker, K. B., Mazurek, M. O., & Hathaway, S. L. (2006). Masculine role adherence and outcomes among men with traumatic brain injury. *Brain Injury, 20,* 1155–1162. doi:10.1080/02699050600983735

Simpson, G., Simons, M., & McFadyen, M. (2002). The challenges of a hidden disability: Social work practice in the field of traumatic brain injury. *Australian Social Work, 55*(1), 24–37. doi:10.1080/03124070208411669

Teasdale, G. (1995). Head injury. *Journal of Neurology, Neurosurgery and Psychiatry, 58,* 526–539.

Teasdale, G., & Jennett, B. (1976). Assessment and prognosis of coma after head injury. *Acta Neurochirurgica, 34*(1–4), 45–55. doi:10.1007/bf01405862

Thomas, J., & Harden, A. (2008). Methods for the thematic synthesis of qualitative research in systematic reviews. *BMC Medical Research Methodology, 8,* 45–55. doi:10.1186/1471-2288-8-45

Wagner, A. K., Sasser, H. C., Hammond, F. M., Wiercisieswski, D., & Alexander, J. (2000). Intentional traumatic brain injury: Epidemiology, risk factors, and associations with injury severity and mortality. *The Journal of Trauma: Injury, Infection, and Critical Care, 49,* 404–410. doi:10.1097/00005373-200009000-00004

Wenden, F., Crawford, S., Wade, D., King, N., & Moss, N. (1998). Assault, post-traumatic amnesia and other variables related to outcome following head injury. *Clinical Rehabilitation, 12*(1), 53–63. doi:10.1191/026921598675567949

Wheeler, S., Accord-Vira, A., & Davis, D. (2016). Effectiveness of interventions to improve occupational performance for people with psychosocial, behavioral, and emotional impairments after brain injury: A systematic review. *American Journal of Occupational Therapy, 70,* 7003180060p1–7003180060p9. doi:10.5014/ajot.115.020677

World Health Organization Global Consultation on Violence, & Health. (1996). *Violence: A public health priority.* Geneva, Switzerland: World Health Organization.

Zafonte, R., Mann, N., Millis, S., Black, K., Wood, D. L., & Hammond, F. (1997). Posttraumatic amnesia: Its relation to functional outcome. *Archives of Physical Medicine and Rehabilitation, 78,* 1103–1106. doi:10.1016/s0003-9993(97)90135-0

A Clarion Call for Social Work Attention: Brothers and Sisters of Persons With Acquired Brain Injury in the United States

Charles Edmund Degeneffe

ABSTRACT

This article presents a clarion call for increased social work attention to the needs of siblings of persons with acquired brain injury (ABI) in the United States. The article overviews how siblings are psychosocially affected, how they provide care to the injured brothers and sisters, and how they personally develop as a result of their experiences. The article highlights the fact that social workers and other professionals often overlook the needs of siblings of persons with ABI and makes an appeal for social workers to advance clinical practice and research to benefit this often neglected population.

Sometimes referred to as a silent epidemic, acquired brain injury (ABI) presents a significant public health care challenge in the United States and other countries throughout the world. Although the silent epidemic moniker remains associated with ABI, professional and public consciousness grows about the serious, and at times profound, consequences of ABI on injured persons, reducing the relevance of the "silent" idiom. In the United States, for example, the recent release of the motion picture *Concussion* highlights the impacts of repeated blows to the head experienced among professional football players, such as a brain disease termed *chronic traumatic encephalopathy*. Also, long-standing participation in Operation Enduring Freedom (OEF) and Operation Iraqi Freedom (OIF) by the United States and its allies highlights the impacts of polytrauma injuries incurred by military personnel subject to improvised explosive devices.

ABI refers to the overall category of brain injury and is categorized in terms of traumatic versus nontraumatic forms of injury. Traumatic brain injury (TBI) occurs from brain injury resulting from an external force to the head and can occur regardless of whether the skull and meninges are intact (i.e., closed head injury) or fractured (i.e., open head injury). According to the Centers for Disease Control and Prevention (CDC, 2016), from 2006 to

2010, the leading cause of TBI in the United States was falls (40.0%) followed by unintentional blunt force trauma (15.5%), motor vehicle accidents (14.3%), and assaults (10.7%). Another 19.0% of TBIs are due to unknown or other causes. Nontraumatic forms of ABI include such examples as strokes, surgical accidents, and aneurisms. It is estimated that approximately 795,000 Americans annually will incur nontraumatic ABIs (Roger et al., 2012) and 1.7 million will become injured through TBI (Faul, Xu, Wald, & Coronado, 2010). About 50,000 Americans die from TBI annually (CDC, 2015).

Although awareness about ABI continues to increase, the many family implications of ABI are not as well known. Modern medicine offers an incredible array of acute and inpatient interventions following ABI, which provide injured persons a much higher chance of survival than in previous years. However, following acute-care services, there is a large drop-off in professional attention to the long-term needs of persons with ABI. The range and availability of long-term services to meet the chronic needs of persons with ABI is largely insufficient and differs widely among geographical locations and disability systems. Families therefore face long-term and extended caregiving responsibilities, often with little to no support, as they work to meet the lifelong needs of their injured family members.

Over the past 20 years, researchers have investigated the many ways that families are affected post-ABI with regard to family system changes, the outcomes of caregiving-related stresses, and the manner in which family members adjust their lives to provide care. Most of the available research focuses on spouses or partners (e.g., Bodley-Scott & Riley, 2015; Knox, Douglas, & Bigby, 2015a) or parents (e.g., Knox, Douglas, & Bigby, 2015b; Raj et al., 2015). On the surface, this is not surprising. Spouses or partners and parents are likely to be the primary points of contact during acute-care services, given their ability to make health care decisions. They are the family members best able to provide information to hospital staff on insurance, the health history of the injured family member, and their anticipated role as primary caregivers following discharge. Spouses or partners and parents will therefore be the family members most accessible to researchers who frequently recruit samples through their contact with hospital staff or the membership rolls of ABI support organizations.

On further examination, however, a major shortcoming in professional understanding of family response to ABI concerns siblings. For the same reasons that studies primarily focus on spouses or partners and parents, the lack of a sibling focus likely occurs because siblings lack contact with clinical treatment staff, and are therefore not as easily accessible to researchers. The term *silent* is a term that better applies to this family subgroup. This lack of professional attention is unfortunate, given the special relationship siblings maintain with their injured brothers and sisters. Like primary caregivers, siblings are likely to be deeply emotionally affected by a brother's or sister's

ABI. Families sometimes hold expectations for siblings to assume lifelong care responsibilities; siblings can find the direction of their lives suddenly changed due to the unexpected nature of ABI.

Accordingly, the purpose of this article is to serve as a clarion call to social workers on the need to apply specific professional attention in research, clinical practice, and pre- and continuing education to the neglected population of siblings of persons with ABI. Social workers encounter families of persons with ABI (Degeneffe, 2001) through positions as hospital discharge planners, service coordinators for nonprofit agencies supporting persons with ABI, and in agencies providing psychotherapeutic support to families of persons with disabilities. Through these positions, there are many opportunities for social workers to engage with and facilitate the participation of siblings in the rehabilitation process of persons with ABI from childhood throughout the adult years. To advance awareness of the needs and unique experiences of siblings, this article addresses the following areas: (a) family response to ABI; (b) sibling response to ABI; and (c) clinical, policy, and research recommendations.

Family response to ABI

Following ABI, there is a broad range of recovery that can occur among injured persons. Many people with ABI make substantial recovery, psychologically adjust, and engage productively with their social relationships, employment, and community involvement. These factors are related to the injured person's ability to perceive positive quality of life postinjury (Berger, Leven, Pirente, Bouillon, & Neugebauer, 1999; Degeneffe & Lee, 2010). However, others find difficulty maintaining relationships due to an inability to control inappropriate behaviors (Medlar, 1998). Many persons with ABI struggle with returning to work or working at their preinjury capacity (Degeneffe et al., 2008). Some individuals with ABI continually compare their postinjury lives to their preinjury lives and are not able to fully acknowledge their new reality (Prigatano, 1995). Those not able to independently meet their own needs often turn to family for care and support.

For some families, the choice to provide care comes from feelings of loyalty and family commitment (DeJong, Batavia, & Williams, 1990). For other families however, the injured person might have no one else to turn to, given the deficient nature of long-term care for persons with ABI in the United States. The United States enjoys state-of-the-art treatments to respond to ABI at the acute-care stage of rehabilitation, in part informed by advances in battlefield medicine through OEF and OIF operations. However, after discharge, a different picture emerges.

States differ, for example, on public funds devoted to ABI services and participation in the TBI Medicaid Waiver Program, and vary with regard to how ABI is defined for service eligibility (Degeneffe et al., 2008). Even when services are available, what is present might be insufficient. Degeneffe and Tucker (2014) surveyed 28 persons in leadership positions with Brain Injury Association of America (BIA) state affiliate organizations. The leaders indicated that with the exception of sexuality training (70.4%), the percentage of unavailable services in 11 other service categories ranged from 0 to 37.0%, in such areas as supported employment, personal attendant care, and legal services. However, when asked to rate the extent to which available services were adequate in all 12 categories, percentages only ranged from 3.6% to 25.0%.

Family care can be limited to simple tasks such as providing reminders that extend to meeting all the injured person's needs, such as dressing, toileting, and feeding. Because ABI occurs randomly and without warning, family caregivers are not prepared to undertake the challenges of caregiving, as many of these areas require specific training and expertise on knowing how to properly intervene in such areas as sexuality expression, behavior management, medication management, and alcohol and drug abuse (Degeneffe, 2001). This distinguishes family caregiving among persons with ABI from those with disabilities such as intellectual disability, autism, and Alzheimer's disease, where family can have many years to adjust and adapt their family routines, build their caregiving skills, and make life choices consistent with their role as caregiver, such as choices related to career and intimate relationships.

Family stressors can be experienced on system and individual levels. From a family systems perspective, families can change their means of communicating, solving problems, and overall functioning as a family unit. Kosciulek (1996), for example, examined how family adaptation and communication style impacted the family's overall sense of cohesion following TBI for 82 caregivers. As measured on the Family Adaptability and Cohesion Evaluation Scale II, cohesion was higher for families better able to adapt and effectively communicate. To help in managing the various strains and stresses that follow ABI, studies on family response to ABI consistency find families need help with financial advice, medical information, and emotional and social supports (Bishop, Degeneffe, & Mast, 2006).

Unfortunately, the ability and willingness of professionals to meet the various needs of families of persons with ABI can at times be limited to nonexistent (Degeneffe & Bursnall, 2015; Degeneffe & Tucker, 2014; Tucker & Degeneffe, 2013). Many families, not surprisingly, struggle in their response to ABI. Gan, Campbell, Gemeinhardt, and McFadden (2006) found, for example, greater levels of distressed family functioning compared to a normative sample on the Family Assessment Measure–II.

As families experience systemic changes and impacts, family members also individually experience unique stresses and concerns. The uniqueness of family responses to ABI suggests that each member requires tailored support to meet his or her particular needs, which might differ considerably from other family members. Degeneffe's (2001) review highlighted distinctive concerns among parents, children, spouses or partners, and siblings. Parents can disproportionally place attention on the injured family member at the exclusion of attending to their other children. Parents might also try to address previously unresolved preinjury issues with their injured sons or daughters. Children might find themselves in a role reversal of providing care to an injured parent instead of being cared for by the parent. Children can experience embarrassment if their injured parent acts in unusual ways. Spouses and partners might need to shift from an equalitarian relationship to one of making decisions on behalf of a spouse or partner, and encounter difficulty in relating to someone now quite different in personality. Finally, siblings face their own unique set of concerns and stresses as they adjust to their brother's or sister's ABI.

Sibling response to ABI

In their response to ABI, siblings encounter a range of emotions, concerns, and life changes distinct from other family members, which are largely not well known among clinicians and researchers. It can be reasonably assumed that social workers and other ABI professionals believe the impact of ABI on siblings pales in comparison to that on parents and spouses or partners, based on their observation that parents and spouses or partners are the persons assigned primary care responsibilities, and they are able to see firsthand their caregiving-related stresses and strains. In the discussion that follows, however, the available research on siblings counteracts this assumption.

To understand the sibling experience following ABI, it is important to first acknowledge how the sibling relationship differs from other human relationships. The affection and love siblings feel for each other can be more intensely felt than in other relationships due in part to the duration and egalitarian nature of the sibling relationship (Cicirelli, 1991), which often starts in childhood and continues through the process of such life events as going through adolescence, getting married, having children, getting divorced, and grieving the loss of parents. Siblings also share a sense of familiarity and common experience sometimes stronger than any of their other relationships, given a shared family history, genetic background, and cultural and religiously based values and belief systems. One's brother or sister therefore serves as a reflection of the self. Siblings' sense of affiliation can encompass the normative years of childhood to old age (Seltzer, Begun, Seltzer, & Krauss, 1991).

Psychosocial responses to ABI

The bulk of family caregiving research following ABI focuses on documenting how family members are psychologically affected, how families are affected as a system, and how families (as a system) work to psychologically adjust and adapt (McIntyre & Kendall, 2013). A consensus from this research area is that family members often experience high rates of burden, depression, and anxiety on an extended basis, and family systems struggle to function in a healthy and productive manner. These findings are not all that surprising given the many challenges of providing extended care in a context of insufficient community-based supports, with a perception that caregiving responsibilities will continue indefinitely. Also, these findings highlight the difficulty families can encounter in using effective coping strategies and mobilizing social supports (Degeneffe, 2001).

Specific to siblings, the available research suggests that siblings face a range of psychological and emotional reactions extending from childhood to the adult years comparable in intensity to what other family members experience. In the child and adolescent years, research finds that siblings can be negatively psychologically affected (Sambuco, Brookes, & Lah, 2008) in a variety of domains. For example, in a study of 39 siblings closest in age to child siblings with moderate to severe TBI, Sambuco, Brookes, Catroppa, and Lah (2012) found siblings experienced significantly reduced self-esteem (i.e., as measured on the Self-Perception Profile for Children–Global Self-Worth scale). Also, Swift et al. (2003) compared relationship quality between 64 siblings of children with TBI and 39 siblings with orthopedic injuries (not involving TBI). Siblings of a different gender to their brothers and sisters with TBI were found to have more negative relationships compared to siblings in the non-TBI, orthopedic injury group.

Several qualitative studies illustrate the nature of pediatric response to a brother's or sister's ABI. A key finding that emerges from these studies is that ABI disrupts the sibling's childhood sense of safety and normalcy, as they need to adjust to new demands, different parental attention, and a changed relationship to their injured brother or sister. For example, Bursnall (2003) found in a Queensland, Australia, sample of 28 siblings (20 child and adolescent siblings of persons with ABI, 4 adult siblings of persons with ABI, and 4 child and adult siblings of persons with cognitive disabilities) that siblings experienced a lost equilibrium in response to worries about the overall functioning of their families, as well as by the revealing of mortality and the long-term implications of their siblings' ABI. Siblings reported acute anxiety, ongoing worry, grief, ambivalence, and a loss of predictability, safety, security, and control. Bursnall offered the following quote to demonstrate an instance of how an 11-year-old male sibling struggled with observing changes with his injured sister:

> I sometimes feel worried. Sometimes she talks during her sleep and I have no idea why she talks. I have noticed it happening this year and last year, but I don't know. I would know if she had always done that ... I worry about that, I don't know what's going to happen, she starts talking like she's talking to herself like this ... I don't know what's happening ... (And) I worry about her safety. (p. 122)

As found with research on child and adolescent siblings of persons with ABI, studies on adult siblings also find evidence of negative psychological outcomes. Orsillo, McCaffrey, and Fisher (1993) measured psychological distress in 13 siblings of persons with TBI with an average age of 24 years (ages ranged from 14–30 years). Compared to a normative population on the Brief Symptom Inventory, 83% of participants had significantly higher levels of psychological distress (i.e., caseness). In a study of 170 adult siblings of persons with TBI, Degeneffe and Lynch (2006) reported that approximately 39% had scores of 16 or above on the Center for Epidemiological Studies-Depression (CES-D) scale. (Note that all subsequent references to studies specifically on adult siblings of persons with TBI by Degeneffe and his colleagues were based on data drawn from the same data set.) According to Lewinsohn, Seeley, Roberts, and Allen (1997), CES–D scores of 16 or above identify those at risk for clinical depression.

Like siblings in childhood, a sense of security, safety, and normalcy with family functioning for adult siblings can be severely disrupted. Adult siblings, however, can also struggle with fear of the future, especially as it relates to expectations that they will assume a future caregiving role for their injured brothers and sisters. In another study involving the 28 BIA staff in leadership positions, Tucker and Degeneffe (2013) asked participants to report the types of future concerns conveyed by families supported by their respective BIA state affiliate organizations. The chief fear was determining who would assume future caregiving responsibilities once the primary caregivers were no longer able to serve in this role. Adult siblings themselves internalize this fear. Degeneffe and Olney (2008) determined that for a sample of 280 adult siblings of persons with TBI, the second highest endorsed future concern regarded taking on future caregiving responsibility. Siblings were worried about their capacity to take on an enhanced caregiver role and how this would affect their other responsibilities. For example, one participant stated:

> I am the oldest sibling and the only one living in the same city as my brother who has TBI. I have just started a family; my parents—who have been the primary caregivers—are getting older. What will be my role? … I will become the primary caregiver when my parents cannot. I worry how this will affect my family. I would like my other brother and sister to assume some responsibility as well, but I don't know if this will be possible. I also worry about the needs of my TBI brother; what will his future needs be? (p. 245)

Involvement with care

The limited number of studies (Bursnall, 2003; Degeneffe, 2015; Degeneffe & Burcham, 2008; Gill & Wells, 2000; Willer, Allen, Durnan, & Ferry, 1990) that address sibling caregiving after ABI suggest siblings throughout the life span are active participants in providing care and support to their injured brothers and sisters. Sibling involvement is expressed through advocacy and giving both affective and instrumental types of care. Taking on this responsibility requires siblings to change the flow of their daily activities and can necessitate role changes and role reversals. For social workers and other professionals, this might come as a surprise, given their primary contact with parents and spouses or partners during both acute- and long-term-care services. Sibling involvement derives in part from the power of the sibling relationship and the level of commitment siblings direct toward their injured brothers and sisters. There can be psychological benefits for siblings to be involved in the care of their brothers and sisters with ABI. Jacobs (1989) argued that family involvement in the rehabilitation process facilitates feelings of empowerment rather than helplessness postinjury.

Child and adolescent siblings express their involvement through a variety of strategies. Bursnall (2003) noted siblings took on the role of a surrogate parent, where siblings worked in partnership with parents to respond to the needs of their injured family members. The surrogate parent role was expressed in a variety of ways, including, for example, acting as a protector against those who wished to victimize their brothers and sisters with ABI. To illustrate this role, Bursnall offered the following quote from a 13-year-old female sibling:

> Me and mum were waiting in the car for him after school and at the lollipop cross-ing this kid pushed my brother around and called him [names] and I chased after him and I abused the living hell out of him. ... I made it pretty clear to him. ... It happens and you like just want to get revenge for them. (p. 153)

Consistent with a surrogate parent role, Gill and Wells (2000) described how siblings of persons with TBI helped guide their brothers and sisters by offering encouragement, helping them to think through problems, and pro-viding verbal disapproval when their siblings acted inappropriately. Gill and Wells interviewed eight siblings (ranging from 14–30 years old) living with their parents and the family member with TBI. They further discussed how siblings took on different family roles to provide care (e.g., younger sibling taking on the role of being the older brother). In their study of 12 families of young adult males with TBI in Ontario, Canada, Willer et al. (1990) also noted siblings specifically prepared themselves to provide care and advocacy for their brothers and sisters to reengage with preinjury activities and friendships.

Adult siblings likewise engage in caregiving despite not living with their injured brothers or sisters and in many cases, living hundreds of miles away. Degeneffe and Burcham's (2008, pp. 13–14) study on 233 adult siblings of persons with TBI found siblings actively provided a variety of affective and instrumental forms of care despite living on average 189 miles from their injured brothers and sisters. In rank order, siblings provided (a) general support and encouragement, (b) companionship, (c) occasional check-ins, (d) transportation, (e) direct caregiving assistance (including medical care), (f) help running errands, (g) assistance dealing with service providers and agencies, (h) help setting up services, (i) help managing finances, and (j) financial support. The first three types of support were grouped as affective caregiving support and were provided significantly more than the final seven types of supports, categorized as instrumental caregiving support. Not surprising, geographical distance was inversely related to the provision of instrumental care, whereas affective forms of care occurred regardless of proximity. The finding of greater provision of affective care was also found by Seltzer et al. (1991) in their study of adult siblings of persons with intellectual disability.

Although adult siblings are willing to provide care, they might be unprepared to assume greater caregiving responsibilities in future years. In a study of 30 parent and adult sibling dyads of persons with ABI in a large southwestern city in the United States, Degeneffe (2015) found that although many siblings were willing to be a future caregiver for their injured brothers and sisters, they would do so with reluctance. Many parents likewise were reluctant to pass on a future caregiver role to siblings. The disinclination for siblings to engage in future care might be related to the lack of caregiving planning that families had undertaken, due to families not being willing or able to engage in this process. In describing the lack of planning, one sibling commented:

> The question came up about 3 months ago just prior to the invitation to participate in your survey. My father just died recently and I told my mother I was going to call a family meeting regarding my sister's long-term care. My idea was rejected (52-year-old sister; 4 years since injury). (p. 11)

Personal development

As siblings come to terms with a different life in the aftermath of ABI, many experience substantial and life-altering life modifications. On the surface, siblings find their daily activities change as the family works to mobilize around meeting the care needs of the injured family member. Further, siblings find changed relationships not only with their injured brothers and sisters, but likewise with parents, friends, and other family members. On a deeper level, siblings sometimes find a new meaning to their lives with regard to values, priorities, and purpose. Child and adolescent siblings encounter these changes in the context of the many developmental changes they are already experiencing. Adult siblings encounter these changes in the context of lives already defined with regard to children, spouse or partner relationships, and career choices.

A driving force behind the life changes encountered by siblings is that it reflects the ways they attempt to cope with all of the emotions they are processing in their post-ABI adjustment.

In Bursnall's (2003) study of pediatric ABI, she referred to this process as one of *regaining equilibrium,* where siblings engaged in a variety of navigating and sacrificing processes to regain a sense of harmony and homeostasis. *Navigating* involved a set of processes where siblings integrated their new reality by revising the ways they related to family rules and relationships, including such strategies as withdrawing from family interactions, as well as adapting their adjustment strategies until they found what worked best. Bursnall offered the following quote to demonstrate how a 17-year-old male sibling made sense of his new life:

> Because it happened we have got to deal with it. ... You can't really change that. That is who he is now, and accept it and work with it and not against it. ... I mean you have got to work with that and it doesn't matter what you think or how much you cry about it, it is not going to [change]. ... There's no point in saying "if this" or "if that"; it's happened so you have just got to get on with your life. (p. 146)

Gill and Wells (2000) also found siblings redefined their relationships with the injured person and other family members and friends.

The second domain in the Bursnall (2003) regaining equilibrium model, *sacrificing,* referred to strategies where siblings set their own needs and interests below those of the injured brother or sister and other family members, such as giving up expectations for parental attention and repressing their own needs for emotional expression. For example, in explaining why he understood his parents could not give the same attention to all the children, a 13-year-old male sibling stated:

> Mum and dad are like totally even with all of us, give us all the same attention sort of thing. ... Oh I've felt like that [left out] a lot but like I know deep down that I'm not left out at all, like sometimes I feel left out and that I am hard done by, but not a lot. ... When do I most feel left out? When he is sort of getting all the attention, but I don't really feel left out. I know that he needs the attention because that's the way he gets through. (pp. 160–161)

Willer et al. (1990) likewise found a need to repress emotions conveyed by seven siblings (with an average age of 17 years) in structured group discussions. Siblings discussed the necessity of suppressing feelings of frustration and developing patience in response to the challenges presented by their family members' TBI.

Due to changes in their priorities, lifestyles, and relationships post-ABI, siblings of persons with ABI can acquire personal development beyond what would have occurred if no injury had taken place. Bursnall (2003) noted through sacrificing processes, siblings reported perceptions of being more tolerant, cautious, responsible, and understanding. Gill and Wells (2000) likewise found siblings felt they changed their priorities due to their increased caregiving responsibilities, as well as enhanced self-awareness. In describing self-awareness, Gill and Wells stated, "It was a wake-up call prompting them to rethink who they were, what they wanted to do, and why they were doing it" (p. 51).

The types of personal development described by Bursnall (2003), Gill and Wells (2000), and Willer et al. (1990) appear to also occur in adulthood. This is somewhat surprising given that many adult siblings might no longer live with their injured brothers and sisters and can be many years removed from the time of injury. This highlights the pervasive influence of ABI. Degeneffe and Olney (2010) examined how the lives of 272 adult siblings of persons with TBI were changed following injury. The mean age of siblings was 38; they lived an average of 185 miles from their injured brothers and sisters, and resided in 23 different U.S. states and one country outside the United States. On average, siblings were approximately 25 years of age at the time of injury. Degeneffe and Olney identified three domains of life changes: (a) family, (b) caring, and (c) making sense of the experience.

The making sense of the experience (Degeneffe & Olney, 2010) domain addressed the ways siblings psychologically reacted and viewed their lives differently postinjury. Although siblings acknowledged the difficulty of TBI, they also recognized the many positive ways they developed as human beings. With regard to negative responses, siblings discussed grieving the loss of the brother or sister they knew preinjury, feeling psychological distress, and experiencing guilt over not being more involved in their injured siblings' lives. However, siblings also conveyed the powerful ways their lives were changed in a positive manner, such as evaluating and redefining life choices (e.g., careers), values, and priorities. Some siblings also experienced existential insights about the true meaning of their lives. For example, in discussing how his faith in God was strengthened, a 21-year-old male sibling commented:

> I rely more on God to handle my problems than before. I have learned a great deal more about how little I control in my life. I have a greater respect for life and the time that I have here on Earth (Participant 176; 21-year-old male; 1 year since the injury). (p. 1423)

Clinical, policy, and research recommendations

The discussion of sibling response to ABI highlights the need for social workers to provide specific support and attention to this often neglected population. Following ABI, siblings will have a range of questions and concerns, which can easily be overlooked if their involvement is not sought out during acute and long-term support services (Degeneffe, 2015).

For example, in a sample of 158 adult siblings of persons with TBI in the United States, Degeneffe (2009) assessed sibling needs via the Family Needs Questionnaire (FNQ), an instrument that assesses the importance of needs for health information, professional support, instrumental support, involvement with care, emotional support, and being part of a community support network. The FNQ also determines the extent to which these needs have been met. Degeneffe found a high level (73.1%) of need across the six domains, with the need for health information (87.4%) as the highest area of need. However, only 41.9% of needs across the six domains were rated as met.

Clinical interventions

Social workers should tailor their interventions to meet the specific support needs of younger versus older populations. In working with younger siblings of persons with ABI, Bursnall (2013) stressed ABI will be uniquely experienced from sibling to sibling. Accordingly, Bursnall stated, "Therefore, when assisting siblings, one must keep in mind that each person should be listened to carefully and their individual experiences and needs assessed" (p. 109).

Bursnall (2003, 2013) also provided specific suggestions for professional intervention. First, siblings should be assisted to openly express and process their feelings and be given validation that what they are experiencing is normal. Siblings should be given information about their family member's ABI matched to what they can comprehend and emotionally manage. Their contributions and sacrifices on behalf of their families and injured brothers and sisters with ABI should be acknowledged. Siblings need special attention and time with their parents separate from their injured brothers and sisters. Finally, siblings can benefit by hearing from other siblings of persons with ABI about how to adjust and cope.

In the long term, adult siblings require assistance with understanding the life-span implications of their brothers' and sisters' injuries regarding their ability to live independently, work, and maintain their physical and emotional health. Degeneffe's (2015) study of 30 parent–adult sibling dyads highlights the little preparation that siblings receive in getting ready to assume a greater future caregiver role. Social workers are encouraged to proactively facilitate long-term planning discussions with families years before parents or other family members relinquish their primary caregiver role. By doing so, siblings can adjust their future plans to incorporate an enhanced caregiver role, including such decisions as buying a house with room for the injured sibling and working and living in close proximity to their brother or sister. Also, social workers can link siblings with training resources on how to give care in such areas as behavioral management and cognitive rehabilitation.

Siblings should also be given the opportunity to process their feelings of loss experienced in childhood, adolescence, and the adult years. In each of the periods, siblings might grieve the sibling they knew preinjury and what their relationships would have been had no injury occurred to their brother or sister. For example, Degeneffe and Olney (2010) offered the following quote to explicate the nature of grieving reactions in their study of 272 adult siblings of persons with TBI:

> I also felt the loss of a close rapport with my sister; she had been the hero I looked up to, and now our roles were somewhat reversed. Because I am her younger sister, my "milestones" were difficult for her to accept; that I reached them when she hadn't: H.S. graduation, college graduation, marriage and now first child (Participant 172a; 31-year-old female; 17 years since the injury). (p. 1423)

Siblings should be given the opportunity to process these types of losses. Doka (2002) suggested persons in various walks of life are sometimes not allowed to grieve, which Doka referred to as *disenfranchised grief*. Of relevance to siblings of persons with ABI, Doka stated, "That right to grieve may not be accorded for many reasons, such as the ways a person grieves, the nature of the loss, or the nature of the relationship" (p. 5). Because of the nature of the sibling relationship (which often does not involve primary caregiving responsibilities to the same extent as parents and spouses or partners), siblings might feel they do not deserve support for their psychological needs to the same extent as other family members more directly involved in caregiving. Likewise, families might assume the noninjured sibling is not distressed to the same level as other family members more actively involved in caregiving.

Also, because siblings are often in the background and not fully accessible to social workers and other ABI professionals, their psychological needs to address feelings of loss and grief can go unresolved and unrecognized. Boss (1999) referred to feelings of misunderstood and unprocessed loss as *ambiguous loss*. Speaking to the psychological pain of ambiguous loss, Boss noted, "Ambiguous loss is always stressful and often tormenting. Information about it belongs in the literature of psychotherapy as well as in the arts" (p. 5).

Social workers possess a range of interventions to address the psychological and emotional needs of siblings. Efforts should be made to educate other family members about the importance of recognizing the needs of siblings and to incorporate sibling involvement in the care of the injured family member. These efforts can begin during acute rehabilitation. During this phase, it is easy to overlook siblings if they are not in direct contact with ABI professional staff. Specific efforts need to be made to bring siblings into professional interactions such as a physician reviewing the recovery status of the injured person or discharge planning discussions about the injured person returning home. On a longer term basis, social workers can likewise address sibling needs and involvement through community-based support groups or through individual or family-based psychotherapy provided in community agencies. Social workers are advised to locate referral sources to support sibling needs that might go beyond their professional training, such as posttraumatic stress disorder, major depression, or other significant mental health conditions.

As noted several times in this article, sibling and family responses to ABI are not universally negative. Although siblings can experience intense feelings of depression, anxiety, loss, and grieving, they can likewise rise to the challenges of ABI and find their lives enhanced in ways impossible had the ABI not occurred. Siblings can be highly resilient and adaptive to the stresses presented by ABI, and can respond in ways that exceed their perceived capabilities. It is important for social workers and other ABI professionals to recognize and foster these capabilities from a strengths rather than deficiency perspective. Professionals are therefore encouraged to incorporate siblings into interventions to meet the needs of the injured family member, as well as the family as a system.

To effectively follow these practice recommendations, social workers need specific training on ABI beyond what they might get during their formative training. In the United States, the Council on Social Work Education (2012) sets accreditation standards for university programs offering academic degrees in social work. Its current standards fail to mention ABI and only mention disability in the context of diversity. Social workers are advised to learn about ABI and related disabilities through independent study, workshops, and additional training. One option is attaining the Certified Brain Injury Specialist credential from the BIA (2015). Through this training, certificate holders learn about such areas as brain anatomy and brain–behavior relationships, family issues, and the continuum of services. Also, the Rehabilitation Research and Training Center on Community Integration of Persons with Traumatic Brain Injury (2014) offers ABI training specific to social work practice, which includes a PDF document (http://www.brainline.org/downloads/PDFs/SystematicApproachtoSocialWorkPractice.pdf) and online course (http://www.tbicommunity.org/resources/courseAvenue/index.htm).

Policy recommendations

Social workers possess a history of advocating for public policy, legislation, and funding to meet the needs of stigmatized and marginalized populations. Social workers are encouraged to use their skills in advocacy, community organization, and public engagement to improve the poor state of community-based services for persons with ABI and their families in the United States. In expressing this opinion, Degeneffe (2001) argued:

> To address the shortcomings in services, social workers need to advocate at the local, state, and national levels. Through such advocacy, social workers can make policymakers and program planners better understand needs and challenges faced by families affected by TBI. Given their professional experience and proximity to the daily realities of living with TBI, social workers are in an excellent position to advocate for needed services. (p. 265)

It is important to stress that enhanced community services are needed to help persons with ABI and their families through their collective recovery process and maintain access to social work support beyond the acute-care phase. By advocating for a better system of ABI long-term care, child, adolescent, and adult siblings will be more able to provide care to their injured brothers and sisters and not feel the same level of strain as when no professional support is available.

Areas needing advocacy on the federal level in the United States include fully funding the TBI Act, increasing TBI Medicaid Waiver Programs, and motivating the Rehabilitation Services Administration to offer specific training on vocational rehabilitation for persons with TBI (Degeneffe et al., 2008). One mechanism to promote political advocacy is the National Association of Social Workers (2016) Political Action for Candidate Election (PACE) program. PACE could be used, for instance, to promote the election of politicians who recognize the importance of federally funded ABI research and policy targeted to long-term care and family caregiver support.

Research recommendations

Social work researchers are advised to advance our limited understanding of sibling response to ABI. The bulk of the available research has been conducted by researchers from rehabilitation counseling, rehabilitation psychology, psychology, and nursing. With their understanding of family systems, psychotherapy, social policy, and community-based social welfare programs, social work researchers can make important contributions to the extant research. One strategy to facilitate further social-work-based research is to partner with scholars from academic disciplines already engaged in sibling and ABI family research. Such partnerships can use shared areas of expertise needed to more fully understand how siblings respond to ABI.

A key area needing further examination concerns the life-span impact of ABI on siblings. The studies presented in this article provided information on ways that sibling response to ABI differs in pediatric versus adult sibling populations, but no studies exist that track how childhood ABI influences siblings into their adult years. The adult sibling articles referenced to Degeneffe and his colleagues (Degeneffe, 2009, 2015; Degeneffe & Burcham, 2008; Degeneffe & Lee, 2010; Degeneffe & Lynch, 2006; Degeneffe & Olney, 2008, 2010) were based on samples where on average, TBI had occurred when siblings were already adults. It is possible sibling reactions, coping approaches, and future concerns might be different for siblings affected by ABI in their childhood where ABI was part of their formative development. Also, evidence-based research examining ways to intervene with siblings following

ABI is needed. Given their expertise in providing family-based counseling interventions to families in distress, social work researchers are well poised to pursue this line of research.

Conclusion

Siblings of persons with ABI are a population in need of clinical attention and increased research focus. From childhood to the adult years, siblings provide care to their injured brothers and sisters, and their lives are substantially changed because of their involvement. Given their professional expertise, social work clinicians and researchers are encouraged to place increased professional attention on the often overlooked needs of siblings of persons with ABI. It is my hope this article will motivate the social work profession to mobilize around meeting the needs of this population. The focus of this special issue is a step in the right direction.

References

Berger, E., Leven, F., Pirente, N., Bouillon, B., & Neugebauer, E. (1999). Quality of life after traumatic brain injury: A systematic review of the literature. *Restorative Neurology and Neuroscience, 14*, 93–102.

Bishop, M., Degeneffe, C. E., & Mast, M. (2006). Family needs after traumatic brain injury: Implications for rehabilitation counselling. *The Australian Journal of Rehabilitation Counselling, 12*, 73–87. doi:10.1375/jrc.12.2.73

Bodley-Scott, S. E. M., & Riley, G. A. (2015). How partners experience personality change after traumatic brain injury—Its impact on their emotions and their relationship. *Brain Impairment, 16*, 205–220. doi:10.1017/brimp.2015.22

Boss, P. (1999). *Ambiguous loss: Learning to live with unresolved grief.* Cambridge, MA: Harvard University Press.

Brain Injury Association of America. (2015). *Welcome to ACBIS!* Retrieved from http://www.biausa.org/acbis

Bursnall, S. (2003). *Regaining equilibrium: Understanding the process of sibling adjustment to pediatric acquired brain injury* (Unpublished doctoral dissertation). Griffith University, Nathan, Australia.

Bursnall, S. (2013). Assisting siblings when their brother or sister sustains acquired brain injury. In H. Muenchberger, E. Kendall, & J. Wright (Eds.), *Health and healing after traumatic brain injury* (pp. 101–113). Santa Barbara, CA: Praeger.

Centers for Disease Control and Prevention. (2015). *Traumatic brain injury.* Retrieved from http://www.cdc.gov/healthcommunication/toolstemplates/entertainmented/tips/braininjury.html

Centers for Disease Control and Prevention. (2016). *TBI: Get the facts.* Retrieved from http://www.cdc.gov/traumaticbraininjury/get_the_facts.html

Cicirelli, V. G. (1991). Sibling relationships in adulthood. In S. P. Pfeifer & M. B. Sussman (Eds.), *Families: Intergenerational and generational connections* (pp. 291–310). New York, NY: Haworth.

Council on Social Work Education. (2012). *Educational policy and accreditation standards.* Retrieved from http://www.cswe.org/File.aspx?id=13780

Degeneffe, C. E. (2001). Family caregiving and traumatic brain injury. *Health & Social Work, 26,* 257–268. doi:10.1093/hsw/26.4.257

Degeneffe, C. E. (2009). The rehabilitation needs of adult siblings of persons with traumatic brain injury: A quantitative investigation. *Australian Journal of Rehabilitation Counseling, 15*(1), 12–27. doi:10.1375/jrc.15.1.12

Degeneffe, C. E. (2015). Planning for an uncertain future: Sibling and parent perspectives on future caregiving for persons with acquired brain injury. *Journal of Rehabilitation, 81,* 5–16.

Degeneffe, C. E., Boot, D., Kuehne, J., Kuraishi, A., Maristela, F. D., Noyes, J., ... Will, H. (2008). Community-based interventions for persons with traumatic brain injury: A primer for rehabilitation counselors. *Journal of Applied Rehabilitation Counseling, 39,* 42–52.

Degeneffe, C. E., & Burcham, C. M. (2008). Adult sibling caregiving for persons with traumatic brain injury: Predictors of affective and instrumental support. *Journal of Rehabilitation, 74,* 10–20.

Degeneffe, C. E., & Bursnall, S. (2015). Quality of professional services following traumatic brain injury: Adult sibling perspectives. *Social Work, 60,* 19–28. doi:10.1093/sw/swu047

Degeneffe, C. E., & Lee, G. K. (2010). Quality of life after traumatic brain injury: Perspectives of adult siblings. *Journal of Rehabilitation, 76*(4), 27–36.

Degeneffe, C. E., & Lynch, R. T. (2006). Correlates of depression in adult siblings of persons with traumatic brain injury. *Rehabilitation Counseling Bulletin, 49,* 130–142. doi:10.1177/00343552060490030101

Degeneffe, C. E., & Olney, M. F. (2008). Future concerns of adult siblings of persons with traumatic brain injury. *Rehabilitation Counseling Bulletin, 51,* 240–250. doi:10.1177/0034355207311319

Degeneffe, C. E., & Olney, M. F. (2010). "We are the forgotten victims": Perspectives of adult siblings of persons with traumatic brain injury. *Brain Injury, 24,* 1416–1427.

Degeneffe, C. E., & Tucker, M. (2014). Community-based support and unmet needs among families of persons with brain injuries: A mixed methods study with the Brain Injury Association of America state affiliates. In S. M. Wadsworth & D. S. Riggs (Eds.), *Military deployment and its consequences for families* (pp. 293–313). New York, NY: Springer.

DeJong, G., Batavia, A. I., & Williams, J. M. (1990). Who is responsible for the lifelong well-being of a person with a head injury? *The Journal of Head Trauma Rehabilitation, 5,* 9–22. doi:10.1097/00001199-199003000-00004

Doka, K. J. (Ed.). (2002). *Disenfranchised grief: New directions, challenges, and strategies for practice.* Champaign, IL: Research Press.

Faul, M., Xu, L., Wald, M. M., & Coronado, V. G. (2010). *Traumatic brain injury in the United States: Emergency department visits, hospitalizations, and deaths.* Atlanta, GA: Centers for Disease Control and Prevention, National Center for Injury Prevention and Control.

Gan, C., Campbell, K. A., Gemeinhardt, M., & McFadden, G. T. (2006). Predictors of family system functioning after brain injury. *Brain Injury, 20,* 587–600. doi:10.1080/02699050600743725

Gill, D. J., & Wells, D. L. (2000). Forever different: Experiences of living with a sibling who has a traumatic brain injury. *Rehabilitation Nursing, 25,* 48–53. doi:10.1002/j.2048-7940.2000. tb01862.x

Jacobs, H. E. (1989). Long-term family intervention. In D. W. Ellis & A. Christensen (Eds.), *Neuropsychological treatment after brain injury* (pp. 297–316). Boston, MA: Kluwer Academic.

Knox, L., Douglas, J. M., & Bigby, C. (2015a). "The biggest thing is trying to live for two people": Spousal experiences of supporting decision-making participation for partners with TBI. *Brain Injury, 29,* 745–757.

Knox, L., Douglas, J. M., & Bigby, C. (2015b). "I won't be around forever": Understanding the decision-making experiences of adults with severe TBI and their parents. *Neuropsychological Rehabilitation, 26*(2), 1–25.

Kosciulek, J. F. (1996). The circumplex model and head injury family types: A test of the balanced versus the extreme hypotheses. *Journal of Rehabilitation, 62*(2), 49–54.

Lewinsohn, P. M., Seeley, J. R., Roberts, R. E., & Allen, N. B. (1997). Center for Epidemiologic Studies Depression Scale (CES–D) as a screening instrument for depression among community-residing older adults. *Psychology and Aging, 12,* 277–287. doi:10.1037/0882-7974.12.2.277

McIntyre, M., & Kendall, E. (2013). Family resilience and traumatic brain injury. In H. Muenchberger, E. Kendall, & J. Wright (Eds.), *Health and healing after traumatic brain injury* (pp. 57–70). Santa Barbara, CA: Praeger.

Medlar, T. (1998). The sexuality education program of the Massachusetts statewide head injury program. *Sexuality and Disability, 16,* 11–19.

National Association of Social Workers. (2016). *PACE: Building political power for social workers.* Retrieved from https://www.socialworkers.org/pace/default.asp

Orsillo, S. M., McCaffrey, R. J., & Fisher, J. M. (1993). Siblings of head-injured individuals: A population at risk. *The Journal of Head Trauma Rehabilitation, 8,* 102–115. doi:10.1097/00001199-199303000-00010

Prigatano, G. P. (1995). The problem of lost normality after brain injury. *Journal of Head Trauma Rehabilitation, 10*(3), 87–95.

Raj, S. P., Antonini, T. N., Oberjohn, K. S., Cassedy, A., Makoroff, K. L., & Wade, S. L. (2015). Web-based parenting skills program for pediatric traumatic brain injury reduces psychological distress among lower-income parents. *The Journal of Head Trauma Rehabilitation, 30,* 347–356. doi:10.1097/htr.0000000000000052

Rehabilitation Research and Training Center on Community Integration of Persons with Traumatic Brain Injury. (2014). *Training project 3: Training non-specialist healthcare and educational professionals in the needs of persons with TBI and how to adapt services.* Retrieved from http://www.tbicommunity.org/CurrentProjects/T3/index.html

Roger, V. L., Go, A. S., Lloyd-Jones, D. M., Benjamin, E. J., Berry, J. D., Borden, W. B., … Melanie, B. (2012). Executive summary: Heart disease and stroke statistics—2012 update: A report from the American Heart Association. *Circulation, 125,* 188–197. doi:10.1161/cir.0b013e3182456d46

Sambuco, M., Brookes, N., Catroppa, C., & Lah, S. (2012). Predictors of long-term sibling behavioral outcome and self-esteem following pediatric traumatic brain injury. *The Journal of Head Trauma Rehabilitation, 27,* 413–423. doi:10.1097/htr.0b013e3182274162

Sambuco, M., Brookes, N., & Lah, S. (2008). Paediatric traumatic brain injury: A review of siblings' outcome. *Brain Injury, 22,* 7–17. doi:10.1080/02699050701822022

Seltzer, G. B., Begun, A., Seltzer, M. M., & Krauss, M. W. (1991). Adults with mental retardation and their aging mothers: Impacts of siblings. *Family Relations, 40,* 310–317. doi:10.2307/585017

Swift, E. E., Taylor, H. G., Kaugars, A. S., Drotar, D., Yeates, K. O., Wade, S. L., & Stancin, T. (2003). Sibling relationships and behavior after pediatric traumatic brain injury. *Journal of Developmental & Behavioral Pediatrics, 24*, 24–31. doi:10.1097/00004703-200302000-00007

Tucker, M., & Degeneffe, C. E. (2013). Future concerns among families following brain injury in the United States: Views from the Brain Injury Association of America state affiliates. *The Australian Journal of Rehabilitation Counselling, 19*, 135–141. doi:10.1017/jrc.2013.16

Willer, B., Allen, K., Durnan, M. C., & Ferry, A. (1990). Problems and coping strategies of mothers, siblings and young adult males with traumatic brain injury. *Canadian Journal of Rehabilitation, 3*, 167–173.

Support Persons' Perceptions of Giving Vocational Rehabilitation Support to Clients With Acquired Brain Injury in Sweden

Marie Matérne, Lars-Olov Lundqvist, and Thomas Strandberg

ABSTRACT
The aim of this article is to explore the perception of being a support person for clients with acquired brain injury undergoing vocational rehabilitation. Nine support persons, identified by clients with brain injury, were interviewed. Interviews were analyzed using qualitative content analysis, resulting in 3 themes for assisting the client: commitment, adaptation, and cooperation. Within each theme, multiple dimensions were identified, reflecting the complexity of vocational rehabilitation following acquired brain injury. Commitment built on social relations is linked to sustainability of support. The included support persons' role was especially valuable in contexts where adaptation and cooperation were required.

Previous research shows that support is essential for successful return to work (RTW) in people with acquired brain injury (ABI; Forslund, Roe, Arango-Lasprilla, Sigurdardottir, & Andelic, 2013; Gilworth, Eyres, Carey, Bhakta, & Tennant, 2008; Matérne, Lundqvist, & Strandberg, in press; Tomberg, Toomela, Ennok, & Tikk, 2007). However, research about support persons' perceptions of assisting clients with ABI in the vocational rehabilitation (VR) process is limited. The objective of this study is therefore to explore support persons' perceptions of supporting clients with ABI in a successful RTW.

Vocational rehabilitation denotes all efforts to help someone to return to work and remain in work despite disability (Waddell, Burton, & Kendall, 2008). In Sweden, the VR process involves many parties, such as the Swedish Social Insurance Agency, the Swedish public employment service, employers, and the health care system (SOU, Swedish Government Official Report, 2011). The investigation of claims for sickness benefits and the coordination of benefits are the responsibility of the Swedish Social Insurance Agency.

The rehabilitation and VR process in Sweden is a tax-funded service. Employers have the obligation to organize the workplace and work as best they can to meet the rehabilitation needs of their employees with disabilities (Swedish Work Environment Authority, 1977). What the VR process might look like varies from individual to individual. Personal support systems like case management, as seen in the United Kingdom or Australia, for instance, do not systematically exist in Sweden (Clark-Wilson et al., 2016; Lannin, Henry, Turnbull, Elder, & Campisi, 2012).

Acquired brain injury is an umbrella term that includes brain damage from cerebrovascular accidents, infections, tumors, toxins, and traumatic brain injury (Campbell, 2000). ABI can result in cognitive, physical, emotional, or behavioral impairments, leading to permanent changes in functioning, with consequences for all aspects of the person's life, such as the person's ability to return to work (Campbell, 2000). ABI has an annual incidence of about 100 to 300 per 100,000 people of working age in Western countries (Fortune & Wen, 1999). In Sweden, the yearly incidence of people who acquire a brain injury is approximately 45,000 to 50,000 (Kleiven, Peloso, & von Holst, 2003; Lexell, Lindstedt, Sörbo, & Tengvar, 2007).

Clients with ABI who come back to work rate their life satisfaction higher compared with those still unemployed (Jacobsson, 2010; Kendall, Muenchberger, & Gee, 2006). To return to work is a major goal for many persons with ABI (Alaszewski, Alaszewski, Potter, & Penhale, 2007; Johansson & Tham, 2006). However, RTW rarely happens without extensive support. A support system built for the brain-injured person for keeping in contact with the workplace during the transition phase from sick leave back to work is invaluable (Ellingsen & Aas, 2009). It enables continuous follow-up with the person and facilitates interaction between the parties involved in the VR process, such as the person with ABI, the workplace, the rehabilitation clinic, and the social insurance agency (Ellingsen & Aas, 2009). Support from all the parties throughout the VR process is essential for the client to successfully return to work.

Asked to state who is most important for their recovery and motivation, persons with brain injury have indicated that apart from society and employers, close relatives play an important role (Strandberg, 2009). The family is particularly important because clients with ABI need support for a long time after their injury (Strandberg, 2009). Consequently, one study reported that clients with support from family members in their everyday life experienced lower levels of emotional distress compared to clients receiving no family support (Stergiou-Kita, Dawson, & Rappolt, 2011). It has also been found that involving close family members in the everyday life of persons with ABI leads them to experience less emotional distress during the VR process (Hooson, Coetzer, Stew, & Moore, 2013). Furthermore, other informal support, such as from close friends, also plays an important role and studies show that those with support from friends have a higher probability of returning to work compared to those without support from friends (Forslund et al., 2013). This informal support also lasts longer compared to professional support (Willer & Corrigan, 1994).

Although family and friends are vital, other kinds of support provided by vocational services and rehabilitation staff (e.g., social workers cooperating with occupational therapists) are important for the clients' RTW ability. For example, clinicians could explain the impact of treatment interventions and make recommendations, as clients require information about their injury so that they can participate in decisions about their own rehabilitation, sometimes together with family members (Kissinger, 2008; Knox, Douglas, & Bigby, 2013). Another essential issue is to get professional support from clinicians in dealing with psychological problems. This help is also important in the VR process (Hooson et al., 2013).

Social support at work from colleagues and employers is another factor contributing to the brain-injured person's feeling of being understood and accepted (Ellingsen & Aas, 2009). Whereas a previous study reporting clients' experiences of successful RTW (Matérne et al., in press) contributes to qualitative research on the subject, little research has focused on support at the workplace and from other support persons. This study focuses on support persons identified by the clients in our previous study (Matérne et al., in press). No studies focusing on support persons were identified from the previous literature. To date, very little is known about the role of support persons in VR, and it follows that they are an underutilized resource in current VR models as applied by social and health professionals. The aim of this study is to explore the support persons' perceptions of being a support for clients with ABI in the VR process.

Method

In this study, the definition of successful RTW corresponds to the definition used in previous research (Matérne et al., in press), which is to return to previous work or to a new job at least 50% (e.g., 4 hr a day, 5 days a week) for at least 1 year, after brain injury. There is, to the best of our knowledge, no consensus in the literature on what defines successful RTW.

Participants

All participants in this study were support persons for brain-injured clients participating in a previous study and all provided their support for 8 to 14 years (Matérne et al., in press). The participating clients in that study were 5 men and 5 women aged 27 to 55 years, with mild to moderate ABI, who had gone through VR with successful results. The clients were all recruited

Table 1. Characteristics of the included support persons and the clients with acquired brain injury (ABI).

		Support persons (participants)		The clients with ABI		
No.	Sex	Occupation/function	Formal or informal mandate to support the client	Diagnosis	Years since the brain injury	Occupation postinjury
1	F	Employment consultant/coworker	Informal	Stroke	9	Study counselor
2	M	Security coordinator/coworker	Informal	Stroke	13	Registered nurse
3	F	Employer/manager	Formal	Stroke	12	Masseur
4	F	Employer/manager	Formal	Brain tumor	14	School assistant
5	M	Salesperson/coworker	Informal	Stroke	8	Controller
6	M	Social worker at the outpatient unit for patients with ABI	Formal	Stroke	14	Finance assistant
7	F	Occupational therapist at the outpatient unit for patients with ABI	Formal	Subarachnoid hemorrhage	10	Logistician, transportation
8	F	Employed in the same organization/next of kin	Informal	Stroke	9	Controller
9	F	Employer/personnel manager	Formal	Traumatic brain injury (car accident)	11	Information assistant

from an outpatient clinic in a Swedish county. Their main postinjury problem was cognitive impairment. The ABI clients were asked to select a person who had, in their opinion, been the most important support person in their VR process. Nine of the 10 clients identified a support person and gave permission to the researcher to contact this person. The nine support persons were contacted by letter. They all volunteered to participate in this study. Characteristics of the participants and the clients are shown in Table 1.

The study was approved by the regional ethical review board in Uppsala, Sweden. Written informed consent was obtained from the participants before the interviews.

Procedure

An interview guide was designed by formulating interview questions to address the aim of the research (Kvale & Brinkmann, 2009). Semistructured interviews were chosen because the researcher wanted the participants to talk freely within a structure (Kvale & Brinkmann, 2009; Richards & Morse, 2013). The interviews were performed with the intention to learn more about the support persons' perceptions of giving support in the VR process.

The interview guide consisted of four key areas, which covered (a) the support person's background, (b) the consequences of work for the brain-injured client from the support person's point of view, (c) working life for the client, and (d) support. The interview questions were piloted with a human resource officer before the data collection started. No modification was made to the interview guide after this interview. The participants were free to decide where the interview should take place. Eight of the interviews were conducted in the researcher's office and one in the support person's home. Each interview lasted 60 to 90 min. All interviews were conducted by the first author, and were audio-recorded and transcribed.

The topic of the study, perception of VR, was not that complex for the participants. If unsure of a participant's statement, the interviewer checked with the participant during the interview to clear up any misunderstandings. The material obtained from the 9 participants was rich and included statements covering 225 pages, with the participants having no problem expressing their thoughts on the subject.

Analysis

A hermeneutic approach has been used as a theory of science in this study. This scientific approach provides an interpretation and understanding of texts and aims to reach an understanding of the life-world of an individual or a group of individuals (Gadamer & Lewis, 1997). For analysis of the data, qualitative content analysis was conducted (Graneheim & Lundman, 2004). This method was chosen because it is focused on texts and is suitable for analysis of sensitive and multifactorial phenomena with a distinct research question (Elo & Kyngäs, 2008). Content analysis can capture variations in the interview texts, highlighting similarities and differences, which was considered an advantage in this study. In this study, an inductive approach was used for open-minded examinations and transparency, because there are no previous studies dealing with this phenomenon (Elo & Kyngäs, 2008). The data were structured using the qualitative software program NVivo10 (QSR International, Inc., Cambridge, MA).

The analysis, described by Graneheim and Lundman (2004), consisted of seven steps. The first step started with creating meaning units from a meaningful part of the text. The second step was to condense the meaning units. In the third step, the condensed meaning units were coded with a label. Several codes with similar content were formed into subcategories in the fourth step; these were combined, in the fifth step, into categories. This fifth step was on a manifest and descriptive level. Several categories together formed the sixth step with subthemes, which was on a latent level. In the seventh, and final, step, subthemes are formed into themes, which describe the latent content. The whole analysis process was conducted by the first author and discussed with the second and third authors. In the last two steps, all authors first worked individually and then discussed the findings until consensus was reached about the subthemes and themes. Consensus in this study was a group process in which the input from the three authors was carefully considered, based on listening to each other, to reach an agreement and make a decision on which subthemes and themes best represented the text. No triangulation to validate the findings was conducted.

Results

The data analysis resulted in three themes that described the support person's perception of being a VR support to a client with ABI. The themes were commitment, adaptation, and (c) cooperation. Each theme consisted of three subthemes (see Table 2). The themes are discussed next.

Commitment

The first of the three themes concerns commitment. All participants talked about the importance of commitment from different perspectives. They described their commitment to the client and to the client's VR process and the impact this commitment had for the client's successful RTW. The support persons' commitment meant being a part of the VR process and being involved in the client's working life.

Table 2. Findings divided into themes, subthemes, and categories.

Themes	Subthemes	Categories
Commitment	Supporting the client's motivation and drive	Motivation and drive Poor support gives no result
	The support person's role and empathy	Support from the environment Supporting strategies of support persons Stress and high standards are a barrier for successful RTW
	Support from the workplace	The support person's role is to be a discussion partner, ensure continuity, and provide encouragement
Adaptation	Social and professional skills as adaptation	Skills and social skills are important personal characteristics Reintegration provides confidence
	Adaptation of the client's working conditions	Adaptation of working conditions RTW according to own ability Adaptation of working time
	Adaptability of the workplace and working environments	Workplaces are more difficult to adjust to after a brain injury It is easier to adapt large workplaces on the open labor market
Cooperation	Clear responsibility for the client	Information and communication Economy and certificates can be cumbersome to explain
	Return to the same workplace Coordination of the VR process	Return to the same job is a success factor Cooperation is a key factor Clear organization and accountability are important

Note: RTW = return to work; VR = vocational rehabilitation.

Supporting the client's motivation and drive

One of the three subthemes concerned support as a motivation and drive for the client. The support persons perceived that it was easier for the client to return to work if they themselves were motivated. Lack of commitment on the part of the support person was perceived to negatively affect the client's motivation and consequently also his or her chances to return to work. The participants believed that they played an important role in keeping the client motivated and all of them considered themselves to be highly committed in their support.

The support persons also thought that reasonable demands on the work tasks set by the employer and colleagues were important for the client's motivation. To be a support in the process of setting reasonable demands, the support persons believed that they and the employer first and foremost needed information about the client's condition with respect to the brain injury. With adequate information, it was easier for the support person, the employer, and the client's colleagues to set reasonable demands and be committed to, and supportive in, the client's VR process. One support person described a motivated client who also had managers that set reasonable demands on the client: "Well, partly I think it's this particular motivation and incentive … I also think that the bosses somehow, actually adapted and made just enough demands" (Interviewee 9).

The support person's role and empathy

Another subtheme within this theme of commitment was that of the support person's role. The description the participants gave of their role included "sowing the seeds" for finding new avenues and opportunities for the client in the work situation. Participants further believed that their function as a sounding board and a discussion partner was important. One of the participants described his role as follows:

> I've been an important person, and I've given him a sense of security and calm, and have sort of been able to confirm him. He's been able to communicate this apprehensiveness … to me, so I've been a sort of security filter for him. (Interviewee 6)

An important component of their role as support person was, according to all the participants, the ability to empathize with the client's situation. One support person had personal experience of being seriously ill herself. She felt that she understood the client better; she had a natural commitment for the task, and could easily put herself in the client's situation with feelings of empathy. She felt that her own illness and experience of successful RTW helped her in supporting the client.

> But of course, if you experience a serious health event, like I'd developed breast cancer, obviously your life changes considerably. That's what you hold on to—to friends and to your day-to-day life—in a whole new way. … You understand what it's like when you get some extremely serious disease. (Interviewee 1)

Support from the workplace

Another subtheme that emerged was the importance of support from the working environment. All the support persons emphasized the importance of support from colleagues and others involved in the VR process. The participants talked about commitment at the workplace. Seven of the participants described the important role of acting as a communicator between the client, and his or her colleagues and managers. They highlighted the support from managers as invaluable in successful RTW. One of the participants said that the manager was unsupportive and not sufficiently committed, so the client lost motivation for RTW.

> I mean, you've got to admit X recovered extremely well, but [he] is naturally dealing with the effects of this stroke as well as the first one … and lost his forward momentum. If you're not getting any support from management either, you lose a great deal of your drive. (Interviewee 2)

In some workplaces, it was natural to help each other; several of the participants had experienced this. For instance, one support person gave an example of a workplace that she thought did not support the client enough; the employer resumed an old conflict when the client came back to work after her sick leave. This support person felt that the employer had no sense of empathy at all. It became quite turbulent at the workplace and the client had a bad start to her RTW. Another participant who worked in a logistics company said that his workplace was committed to solving problems and trying to help each other in different ways. He felt that his colleague's brain injury was regarded at the workplace as just another problem to solve. The support person felt that his role in his colleague's VR process was no different from his normal work as a problem solver. It was like a challenge for him and the workplace to support the client.

> We're actually very used to it, because many people at work here are problem solvers. … That's actually a large part of what we do [solve problems]. So for us it's just another thing to tackle. (Interviewee 8)

Adaptation

The second theme was adaptation. Adaptation, according to the support persons, was about the client's social and professional capacity to adapt, the adaptation of the client's working conditions, and the workplace's potential to adapt the environment that could help the client to manage working life.

Social and professional skills as adaptation

One aspect of adaptation of the client's skills is the social competence several of the participants observed in the brain-injured persons. They defined the client's social competence as the skill to communicate and interact with others, both verbally and nonverbally. These abilities helped the client in his or her RTW. Social skills helped the person with ABI to be accepted more readily in the working group and also to get help with work tasks from colleagues.

Another kind of adaptation that some participants talked about as important was the client's professional competence. Those support persons who assisted clients with extensive professional knowledge and skills facilitated the employer's task to adapt the clients' work tasks because the more skilled and knowledgeable the brain-injured person, the wider the work assignment area: "Involve X in the issues that I know he's really good at, so he feels he can continue working and focusing on issues about which he is knowledgeable" (Interviewee 2).

Adaptation of the client's working conditions

All participants gave examples of different kinds of adaptations for the client at work, ranging from adapted work tasks to completely different work. For example, one participant described a client who worked with children in a preschool. She could not handle the noise and messy environment after her brain injury. Her employer offered her a new job as an administrator for the preschool. Describing an open-minded employer who tried to adapt the work situation for the client, another support person said:

> Yes, it's partly that they are extremely helpful—they want things to go well for the client and are open to change … not just during rehabilitation, but also later on the job—there'll be certain things this person doesn't have to do. (Interviewee 7)

Four of the participants thought that there was a big difference between public and private employers with regard to the possibilities to adapt the working situation. One participant who also was an employer in a public-sector company argued that it was much easier for public-sector companies to make adaptations, both in terms of working time and in terms of performance, compared to companies in the private sector. This employer accepted that the employee did the best she could, without any pressure at all. Another participant with the same experience argued that public companies accept more gradual change and do not have the same financial pressure as companies in the private sector: "It's probably an organization that is not exposed to competition. … I'm not saying it's like, 'Here we are with our quill pens,' but you're not seeing new accounting software every year" (Interviewee 6).

Adaptability of the workplace and working environment

One support person who was the employer of a person with ABI proposed that it has become much harder to adapt the working conditions compared to a few years ago. Her experience was that previously, employers could be more tolerant with people who did not perform their duties quickly or well enough. She thought that the cyclical implication, taking into account the economic situation, of this for adaptation affected the possibilities to return to work and also became a societal problem in the end: "But it's super strict now. It's back to the job you had before. ... So I've had people [employed] after X who have had other concerns and I haven't been able to help them in the same way, it's tough" (Interviewee 4).

Several participants gave examples of how the labor market has become more demanding, saying that it has become easier for employers to dismiss staff members who cannot perform the tasks for which they were hired. This applies to both the private and the public sector. One support person who had met several persons with brain injury at her workplace described that her perception was that workplaces sometimes do not have any willingness at all to cooperate in terms of adaptation or finding new work tasks for a brain-injured employee: "I've been at workplaces where their attitude is, if you can't manage these tasks, we haven't got anything [for you to do]. There's no room for any kind of adaptation" (Interviewee 7).

Another support person, who was the owner and manager of a small family business, made adaptations immediately and developed the business based on the needs that she saw the client had. She had the mandate to make decisions about all kinds of customizations, for example, relating to working time, workloads, and assignments for the client: "So, the organization we had then was amazing; it was such an inspiration for her to feel she was free to do what she wanted, so she has really grown with that" (Interviewee 3).

Cooperation

The third theme was cooperation, which the participants described as an overall collective action on the organizational level to plan for a successful RTW for a client. This organizational level includes authorities who are involved in the VR process for the client. This theme also included cooperation at the workplace among the employer, colleagues, and the client.

Clear responsibility for the client

In the VR process, there has to be cooperation among several government agencies, employers, and the client to create a successful RTW. Talking about cooperation, 7 of the participants emphasized clarity regarding the different parties' roles in the VR process; without clarity, there could be confusion about who does what. The participants gave examples of when the cooperation did not work because of uncertainties between the parties. For example, when there is a change in management, information about the client can get lost and the new manager might not have sufficient information about the client to make decisions about adaptations.

With knowledge about the client's abilities and inabilities, there is increased cooperation among the parties involved in the VR process. Knowledge about the client's needs and disability facilitates cooperation: "I believe information is quite important ... who is supposed to know? How are we going to follow it up? New people coming and going, it's a matter of integrity and consideration for the individual" (Interviewee 9).

Return to the same workplace

Eight of the participants had experience of supporting clients returning to the same workplace as before the injury. Four of the clients also returned to the same duties they held preinjury; this signified success on the part of the clients. One of the participants described that the previous work of a client with ABI had been in economics, but that, after the injury, he experienced problems with numbers and had to change work. With cooperation among the client, the social worker (from the outpatient unit for clients with ABI), and the employer, they found work with new assignments. In this case, it was a job that the client had done previously and could still perform with modifications. Another participant described her client's return to the previous work as follows:

> Partly [the fact] that he could return to his own job, and [partly] that he as a person had a good ground to stand on. ... Going back to work is tough, but in some way, it's what he has done [because] he's familiar with the work, he's used to the working conditions. (Interviewee 9)

Coordination of the vocational rehabilitation process

In the participants' views, those who are involved in the VR process (e.g., employers, the authorities, and outpatient unit staff such as social workers and occupational therapists) all have to coordinate directly with each other to enable the client to reach the goal of returning to work. The cooperation should start soon after the injury, and should include the professionals, as one participant argued:

> It's important to be there and give early support, and that you get professional help and figure out with the [client] ... what I can manage, what I will be able to manage, and how much I should be able to manage now? Support in that process! (Interviewee 2)

Discussion

The aim of this study is to explore support persons' perceptions of supporting clients with ABI in achieving a successful RTW. The analysis elicited three themes that described what the support persons perceived as important for the client to successfully return to work: commitment, adaptation, and cooperation. All support persons testified their commitment to the client. They perceived their role to be vital for the client, especially where adaptation and cooperation were required.

The results show that the support persons' commitment was a factor in helping create and sustain the clients' motivation in the VR process. Also, support and commitment from colleagues and managers at the workplace played a significant role for a successful RTW. However, we found that the ability of support persons, colleagues, and managers to give support was dependent on adequate knowledge about the client's conditions and needs, which is consistent with findings from other studies (Gilworth et al., 2008). Lack of support from the work environment created low client motivation for RTW and also lower commitment from the support person. So it could be hypothesized that one of the key factors to successful RTW is to ensure that adequate support is combined with commitment to create highly motivated clients. This hypothesis is in line with findings by Bonneterre and colleagues that workplace support is a key factor for job retention (Bonneterre et al., 2013).

Previous research shows that support through job coaches, supportive coworkers, or employers with a personal experience of disease or disability could be important for the motivation and ability of workers with ABI to sustain employment (Macaden, Chandler, Chandler, & Berry, 2010). This is consistent with the findings of this study. In our study, one participant reported that she herself had experienced a disease and the subsequent struggle to return to work. She believed that she was better able to understand the client's situation and had become more committed in the client's VR process because of her own personal experience. The results therefore suggest that designating a support person who himself or herself has a personal experience of work rehabilitation could be a favorable approach for supporting clients with ABI to successfully return to work. If it is not possible to find a colleague with a personal experience of work rehabilitation, a coworker could function as a mentor and give support, including support in productivity and self-esteem (Target, Wehman, Petersen, & Gorton, 1998).

Previous research shows that continuity and long-term support are necessary because recovery from ABI takes a long time (van Velzen, van Bennekom, van Dormolen, Sluiter, & Frings-Dresen, 2011). In this study, the participants had given support to the brain-injured persons for 8 to 14 years. As the complexity and difficulty of work tasks change during recovery, a person with ABI needs to have someone close to discuss these issues with during the whole VR process and also for a long time afterward. Where the client can choose the support person himself or herself and build a social relationship with this person, this facilitates and sustains the work for a longer time (Matérne et al., in press).

When the clients in our previous study were asked to choose the most supportive person, they all chose people in the near surroundings, persons at work, relatives, or professionals from the outpatient unit for ABI patients. Only three chose a person with a formal responsibility for client support. It can be concluded that an important support person is not necessarily a person with formal power to act in the rehabilitation process. Much more important is that this person should have a focus on the support, as a discussion partner; for example, helping in the decision-making process for the client (Knox et al., 2013). The interviewed support persons also gave the client confirmation, acted as facilitator for the client at work in different ways, informed colleagues of the client's needs, and understood the client's difficulties. All these actions from the support persons to facilitate the VR process contributed to the successful VR and a sustainable working life for the clients.

Research also shows that it is easier for the client to return to the workplace if he or she is socially accepted by his or her colleagues and managers, because he or she will then receive help if needed (Shames, Treger, Ring, & Giaquinto, 2007). Social skills are, in other words, an important factor for the possibility to return to work. The support persons in this study played an important role in the development of the clients' social skills. A brain-injured person has trust and confidence in his or her support person and together they can reflect on his or her social capabilities.

A workplace often has to adapt work tasks for the client to return after brain injury. The client's professional skills play a key role in this adaptation. Previous studies have suggested that people with white-collar jobs and higher education have better opportunities for job adaptation, contributing to an easier RTW process, compared to their blue-collar counterparts (Kassberg, Prellwitz, & Larsson Lund, 2013; Keyser-Marcus et al., 2002; Walker, Marwitz, Kreutzer, Hart, & Novack, 2006). One of the participants in this study, who herself was a manager and could make decisions about the work situation for the client, adapted the client's work all the time and took into account the disability the client had. This is also in line with Van Velzen et al. (2011), who found the most success occurs if the decision-making process takes place near, and includes, the client. Similarly, in this study, the support persons played an important role in this adaptation process by acting as discussion partners and thus helping to find new opportunities for developing or adapting the client's work tasks.

Cooperation in the VR process is likewise important for a successful RTW. Returning to the preinjury workplace appears to be the best option for a successful RTW. This is in line with findings by Tate, Simpson, and McRae (2014), who argued that the client has already established a relationship with the employer at the preinjury workplace, which facilitates RTW. Furthermore, he or she feels supported in returning to an existing social network at the workplace. Also, returning to a known situation minimizes the need for new learning. Our findings support this. We also found that the employer of a client returning to a known situation is emotionally involved and has more knowledge of the client's competence, which facilitates cooperation in the VR process. Consequently, going back to the preinjury workplace seems to reduce the client's anxiety about the VR process and as a result gives better possibilities for employer–employee cooperation (Tate et al., 2014).

The participants in this study had different kinds of assignments as support persons. Some had a formal mandate as support persons, whereas others acted in a more informal capacity. Regardless of having a formal or an informal mandate, the participants stated that their powers regarding the employer–employee cooperation were unclear. The support persons perceived that nobody is fully in charge of the collaboration, which creates a lack of clarity for all involved, not least the client. The Swedish Social Insurance Agency has a responsibility for coordination, but the assignment is in fact unclear (Ekberg, Eklund, & Hensing, 2015). Vestling, Ramel, and Iwarsson (2013) found that a personal mentor can help the client to return to work. We also found this, but emphasize that this mentor should be well aware of the consequences of the client's brain injury and should be given mandate in the VR process. Despite the fact that the included support persons had different mandates, missions, roles, gender, age, and work, we found that their perceptions of support to the client were comparatively equal.

Study reflections

This study is exploratory and describes the support persons' perceptions of the VR support they gave persons with ABI. However, the results are limited in terms of generalizability to the population of support persons, as we only had 9 participants. The participants in this study had different types of occupations, client relationships, mandates (formal or informal), and working roles, which provided a heterogeneous group and rich material. This is an advantage in a qualitative study that aimed to study differences in the results. All the participants came from a limited geographical area in Sweden, which could give a smaller cultural difference in the group. However, in this study, the clients themselves selected the support persons who were interviewed, which adds interest from a client participation perspective. The group that the support persons in this study supported have mild to moderate ABI, which could, in part, explain the successful RTW outcomes. The situation for persons with severe ABI would be quite different; for instance, more extensive support systems would be required, particularly formal or structured VR service delivery. Therefore, it was not possible to generalize our findings to persons with severe ABI.

Participants in research can change their stories from one telling to the next as a consequence of memory recall. Furthermore, new experiences cause them to see the nature of, and connection between, the events in their lives differently from one time to the next (Sandelowski, 1993). Some years had passed by, but all the participants still had contact with the client; six continued being a support person to the client even at the time of the interviews. The aim was to study the participants' perception, and we captured their opinions about their work as support persons. Therefore, the memory of what it was like to be a support for these participants could be kept alive and the risk of forgetting important events in the VR process was lower than if they had completely lost contact with the clients.

It is important to ensure the validity of the research, which in this study was done by designing the interview questions and study method (Richards & Morse, 2013). The intent was not to verify that data were labeled and sorted in exactly the same way, but to determine whether the researchers agreed with the way those data were labeled and sorted (Woods & Catanzaro, 1988).

To preserve the meanings of the quotes, a language editing company made an initial translation from Swedish to English. This was then reviewed by the authors, with some minor corrections being made to the quotes in discussion with the translator.

Future research

This study explores the support persons' perceptions. One further question that arises is how other parties perceive the VR process. How can the different parties, such as employees, the social insurance agency, or rehabilitation clinics, interact with each other to achieve the best outcome in the VR process for the client? Furthermore, it is interesting to know more about the clients' participation in their own VR, because, as we found in this study, the clients' participation was perceived as a main factor for successful VR. Another research issue concerns the role of VR service provision in Sweden. There is no formal or consistent implementation of VR in Sweden, and the participants in this study raised the matter of lack of role clarity and leadership in the VR process. This area needs more attention to provide a better understanding of the role and contribution that VR services can or could make to the VR process.

Conclusion

Support persons are important to clients with ABI for successfully returning to work. To be chosen by the client to be a support person, with or without a formal mandate, created a commitment. The support persons further perceived that they could be of help in situations that required both adaptation and cooperation. There are many complex and strategic issues that emerge for clients during the VR process that require reflection and decision making. In these situations, the support persons perceived that they were fulfilling an important role. The support person role is often an underutilized resource and could be used systematically in the VR process for clients with ABI.

Acknowledgments

We extend our thanks to the interviewees who participated in this study.

Funding

This study was supported by grants from the University Health Care Research Center, Region Örebro County, Sweden; the Swedish Stroke Association; and the Norrbacka-Eugenia Foundation.

References

Alaszewski, A., Alaszewski, H., Potter, J., & Penhale, B. (2007). Working after a stroke: Survivors' experiences and perceptions of barriers to and facilitators of the return to paid employment. *Disability and Rehabilitation, 29,* 1858–1869. doi:10.1080/09638280601143356

Bonneterre, V., Pérennou, D., Trovatello, V., Mignot, N., Segal, P., Balducci, F., ... de Gaudemaris, R. (2013). Interest of workplace support for returning to work after a traumatic brain injury: A retrospective study. *Annals of Physical and Rehabilitation Medicine, 56,* 652–662. doi:10.1016/j.rehab.2013.10.001

Campbell, M. (2000). *Rehabilitation for traumatic brain injury: Physical therapy practice in context.* Edinburgh, UK: Churchill Livingstone.

Clark-Wilson, J., Giles, G. M., Seymour, S., Tasker, R., Baxter, D. M., & Holloway, M. (2016). Factors influencing community case management and care hours for clients with traumatic brain injury living in the UK. *Brain Injury, 30*(7), 1–11. doi:10.3109/02699052.2016.1146799

Ekberg, K., Eklund, M., & Hensing, G. (2015). Kunskapsbaserade åtgärder för att främja arbetsförmåga och återgång i arbete [Knowledge based measures to promote workability and return to work]. In K. Ekberg, M. Eklund, & G. Hensing (Eds.), *Återgång i arbete - processer, bedömningar, åtgärder* (pp. 219–233). Lund, Sweden: Studentlitteratur.

Ellingsen, K. L., & Aas, R. W. (2009). Work participation after acquired brain injury: Experiences of inhibiting and facilitating factors. *International Journal of Disability Management, 4*(1), 1–11. doi:10.1375/jdmr.4.1.1

Elo, S., & Kyngäs, H. (2008). The qualitative content analysis process. *Journal of Advanced Nursing, 62*(1), 107–115. doi:10.1111/j.1365-2648.2007.04569.x

Forslund, M. V., Roe, C., Arango-Lasprilla, J. C., Sigurdardottir, S., & Andelic, N. (2013). Impact of personal and environmental factors on employment outcome two years after moderate-to-severe traumatic brain injury. *Journal of Rehabilitation Medicine, 45,* 801–807. doi:10.2340/16501977-1168

Fortune, N., & Wen, X. (1999). *The definition, incidence and prevalence of acquired brain injury in Australia.* Canberra, Australia: Australian Institute of Health and Welfare.

Gadamer, H. G., & Lewis, E. H. (1997). *The philosophy of Hans-Georg Gadamer.* Chicago, IL: Open Court.

Gilworth, G., Eyres, S., Carey, A., Bhakta, B. B., & Tennant, A. (2008). Working with a brain injury: Personal experiences of returning to work following a mild or moderate brain injury. *Journal of Rehabilitation Medicine, 40,* 334–339. doi:10.2340/16501977-0169

Graneheim, U. H., & Lundman, B. (2004). Qualitative content analysis in nursing research: Concepts, procedures and measures to achieve trustworthiness. *Nurse Education Today, 24,* 105–112. doi:10.1016/j.nedt.2003.10.001

Hooson, J. M., Coetzer, R., Stew, G., & Moore, A. (2013). Patients' experience of return to work rehabilitation following traumatic brain injury: A phenomenological study. *Neuropsychological Rehabilitation, 23*(1), 19–44. doi:10.1080/09602011.2012.713314

Jacobsson, L. (2010). *Long-term outcome after traumatic brain injury: Studies of individuals from northern Sweden.* Luleå, Sweden: Luleå University of Technology.

Johansson, U., & Tham, K. (2006). The meaning of work after acquired brain injury. *American Journal of Occupational Therapy, 60*(1), 60–69. doi:10.5014/ajot.60.1.60

Kassberg, A.-C., Prellwitz, M., & Larsson Lund, M. (2013). The challenges of everyday technology in the workplace for persons with acquired brain injury. *Scandinavian Journal of Occupational Therapy, 20,* 272–281. doi:10.3109/11038128.2012.734330

Kendall, E., Muenchberger, H., & Gee, T. (2006). Vocational rehabilitation following traumatic brain injury: A quantitative synthesis of outcome studies. *Journal of Vocational Rehabilitation, 25,* 149–160.

Keyser-Marcus, L. A., Bricout, J. C., Wehman, P., Campbell, L. R., Cifu, D. X., Englander, J., … Zafonte, R. D. (2002). Acute predictors of return to employment after traumatic brain injury: A longitudinal follow-up. *Archives of Physical Medicine and Rehabilitation, 83,* 635–641. doi:10.1053/apmr.2002.31605

Kissinger, D. B. (2008). Traumatic brain injury and employment outcomes: Integration of the working alliance model. *Work, 31,* 309–317.

Kleiven, S., Peloso, P. M., & von Holst, H. (2003). The epidemiology of head injuries in Sweden from 1987 to 2000. *International Journal of Injury Control and Safety Promotion, 10*, 173–180. doi:10.1076/icsp.10.3.173.14552

Knox, L., Douglas, J. M., & Bigby, C. (2013). Whose decision is it anyway? How clinicians support decision-making participation after acquired brain injury. *Disability and Rehabilitation, 35*, 1926–1932. doi:10.3109/09638288.2013.766270

Kvale, S., & Brinkmann, S. (2009). *InterViews: Learning the craft of qualitative research interviewing.* Los Angeles, CA: Sage.

Lannin, N., Henry, K., Turnbull, M., Elder, M., & Campisi, J. (2012). An Australian survey of the clinical practice patterns of case management for clients with brain injury. *Brain Impairment, 13*, 228–237. doi:10.1017/BrImp.2012.19

Lexell, J., Lindstedt, M., Sörbo, A., & Tengvar, C. (2007). Farmakologiska möjligheter vid hjärnskadebehandling—Rätt läkemedelsval kan optimera rehabiliteringsinsatserna [Pharmacological possibilities in brain injury rehabilitation]. *Läkartidningen, 104*, 2422–2426.

Macaden, A., Chandler, B., Chandler, C., & Berry, A. (2010). Sustaining employment after vocational rehabilitation in acquired brain injury. *Disability and Rehabilitation, 32*, 1140–1147. doi:10.3109/09638280903311594

Matérne, M., Lundqvist, L.-O., & Strandberg, T. (in press). Opportunities and barriers for successful return to work after acquired brain injury: A patient perspective. *WORK: A Journal of Prevention, Assessment & Rehabilitation.*

Richards, L., & Morse, J. M. (2013). *Readme first for a user's guide to qualitative methods* (Vol. 3.). Los Angeles, CA: Sage.

Sandelowski, M. (1993). Rigor or rigor mortis: The problem of rigor in qualitative research revisited. *Advances in Nursing Science, 16*(2), 1–8. doi:10.1097/00012272-199312000-00002

Shames, J., Treger, I., Ring, H., & Giaquinto, S. (2007). Return to work following traumatic brain injury: Trends and challenges. *Disability and Rehabilitation, 29*, 1387–1395. doi:10.1080/09638280701315011

SOU (Swedish Government Official Report). (2011). *Arbetslivsinriktad rehabilitering rapport nr 7* [Vocational rehabilitation report no. 7] (Vol. 2010:04). Stockholm, Sweden: Statens offentliga utredningar.

Stergiou-Kita, M., Dawson, D. R., & Rappolt, S. G. (2011). An integrated review of the processes and factors relevant to vocational evaluation following traumatic brain injury. *Journal of Occupational Rehabilitation, 21*, 374–394. doi:10.1007/s10926-010-9282-0

Strandberg, T. (2009). Adults with acquired traumatic brain injury: Experiences of a change-over process and consequences in everyday life. *Social Work in Health Care, 48*, 276–297. doi:10.1080/00981380802599240

Swedish Work Environment Authority. (1977). *The Swedish work environment act (1977:1160).* Stockholm, Sweden: Swedish Government.

Target, P., Wehman, P., Petersen, R., & Gorton, S. (1998). Enhancing work outcome for three persons with traumatic brain injury. *International Journal of Rehabilitation Research, 21*, 41–50. doi:10.1097/00004356-199803000-00004

Tate, R., Simpson, G., & McRae, P. (2014). Traumatic brain injury. In R. Escorpizo, S. Brage, D. Homa, & G. Stucki (Eds.), *Handbook of vocational rehabilitation and disability evaluation: Application and implementation of the ICF* (Vol. 2015, pp. 263–294). Cham, Switzerland: Springer.

Tomberg, T., Toomela, A., Ennok, M., & Tikk, A. (2007). Changes in coping strategies, social support, optimism and health-related quality of life following traumatic brain injury: A longitudinal study. *Brain Injury, 21*, 479–488. doi:10.1080/02699050701311737

van Velzen, J., van Bennekom, C., van Dormolen, M., Sluiter, J., & Frings-Dresen, M. (2011). Factors influencing return to work experienced by people with acquired brain injury:

A qualitative research study. *Disability and Rehabilitation, 33,* 2237–2246. doi:10.3109/09638288.2011.563821

Vestling, M., Ramel, E., & Iwarsson, S. (2013). Thoughts and experiences from returning to work after stroke. *Work, 45,* 201–211.

Waddell, G., Burton, A. K., & Kendall, N. A. S. (2008). *Vocational rehabilitation—What works, for whom, and when?* London, UK: TSO.

Walker, W. C., Marwitz, J. H., Kreutzer, J. S., Hart, T., & Novack, T. A. (2006). Occupational categories and return to work after traumatic brain injury: A multicenter study. *Archives of Physical Medicine and Rehabilitation, 87,* 1576–1582. doi:10.1016/j.apmr.2006.08.335

Willer, B., & Corrigan, J. D. (1994). Whatever it takes: A model for community-based services. *Brain Injury, 8,* 647–659. doi:10.3109/02699059409151017

Woods, N. F., & Catanzaro, M. (1988). *Nursing research: Theory and practice.* St. Louis, MO: Mosby.

Social Workers' Perceived Role Clarity as Members of an Interdisciplinary Team in Brain Injury Settings

Martha Vungkhanching and Kareen N. Tonsing

ABSTRACT

This study investigated social workers' role clarity as members of an interdisciplinary team in traumatic and acquired brain injury treatment settings. A total of 37 social workers from 7 Western countries completed an anonymous online survey questionnaire. The majority of participants have more than 10 years of experience working in brain injury treatment settings (59.5%), and about 54% have been in their current employment for more than 10 years. Findings revealed that there were significant positive correlations between perceived respect, team collaboration, and perceived value of self for team with role clarity. Multiple regression analysis revealed that perceived value of self for team was a significant predictor of role clarity ($p < .05$).

Interdisciplinary care is becoming more common today in some areas of geriatric, pediatric, palliative, and rehabilitation health care, and has long been recognized as an important component of effective rehabilitation for persons with traumatic brain injury (TBI; Fordyce, 1981; Prigatano, 1999; Strasser, Uomoto, & Smits, 2008). Terms such as interdisciplinary, multidisciplinary, and transdisciplinary have been commonly used to describe what appear to be very similar forms of care (Barret, Sellman, & Thomas, 2005). Although these three terms are interrelated, they are somewhat different in their approach to working with patients and consumers. In a multidisciplinary team, members with varying skills and experience from different disciplines approach the patient from their own perspective, whereas in a transdisciplinary team, members with different skills and experience from different disciplines transcend their traditional boundaries to come to a consensus about one specific intervention (Choi & Pak, 2006). *Interdisciplinary care* refers to an integrative approach between groups of professionals, including the patient or consumer in a participatory, collaborative, and coordinated approach to shared decision-making around health issues (Orchard, Curran, & Kabene,

2005). The underpinning philosophy guiding interdisciplinary teamwork is that the contribution of each member, with different skills and experience, creates a combined synergy, leading to solutions that are felt to enhance and improve care (Bruner, 1991).

Although the composition of interdisciplinary teams can vary by rehabilitation setting and program, it typically includes representatives of psychiatry, rehabilitation nursing and physicians, speech-language pathology, physical therapy, occupational therapy, social work, neuropsychology or counseling and clinical psychology, and therapeutic recreation. Elements of an effective interdisciplinary team include collaboration, respect for each member's expertise, trust among members, and acceptance and use of each member's style and personal characteristics in the delivery of care (Sander & Constantinidou, 2008; Supiano & Berry, 2013).

As a profession, social work has been involved in collaborating with other disciplines. The social work component in health care has also been noted to increase in importance as the focus on health provision has shifted to incorporate biopsychosocial and holistic approaches (Auslander, 2001). The biopsychosocial model views disease as an interplay among environmental, physical, behavioral, psychological, and social factors. Social work circumnavigates the impact of social, cultural, and economic conditions on health, the impact of illness on personal and family coping, the need for social support, and the importance of multiprofessional collaboration on individual and community health problems (Beddoe, 2011).

TBI is the leading cause of death in individuals under 40 years of age in most Western countries (Keris, Lavendelis, & Macane, 2007), and a major public health issue globally (Smith et al., 2015). According to the Brain Injury Association of America (BIA, n.d.), *acquired brain injury* (ABI) is defined as an injury to the brain that is not hereditary, congenital, degenerative, or induced by birth trauma. This includes brain injuries caused by trauma, stroke, and hypoxia, and excludes brain injuries present at birth or caused by progressive diseases. As one type of ABI, a TBI can be characterized as "an alteration in brain function, or other evidence of brain pathology, caused by external forces" (Menon, Schwab, Wright, & Maas, 2010, p. 1638). The external force can include penetrating injuries (e.g., when an external object pierces the skull and damages brain tissue) or closed head injuries, in which acceleration and deceleration and rotational forces result in the brain colliding with the interior of the skull, resulting in bleeding or bruising of the brain, as well as the shearing of neurons and neuronal tracts (diffuse axonal injury). Common causes of TBI include injury from falls and motor vehicle accidents, as well as from assaults and sporting injuries. All these causes of TBI can result in temporary or permanent changes in physical, mental, and emotional functioning (Moore, 2013). There exists wide variation in the severity of TBI, generally classified as mild, moderate, severe, or very severe (Russell & Smith, 1961).

In the United States, the estimated incidence of TBI is 1.4 million new injuries per year, with approximately 5.3 million individuals living with significant disability as a result of TBI. In Canada, the annual estimated rate of TBI occurrences is 500 per 100,000 individuals (Langois, Rutland-Brown, & Thomas, 2006), and in Sweden, about 450 per 100,000 (Roozenbeek, Maas, & Menon, 2013). In the United Kingdom, an estimated 1 million patients are admitted to the hospital each year following head injury, of which about 5% are severe head injuries (Morris, Ridley, Lecky, Munro, & Christensen, 2008). Findings from a population-based study in New Zealand reported that the total incidence of TBI was 790 cases per 100,000 (Feigin et al., 2013). Based on the findings from a study of management of neurotrauma in Australia, Atkinson and Merry (2001) reported that the number of deaths from head injury was much higher compared to all other deaths. Due to the high rate of people living with significant disability due to their TBI, social workers in health care are very likely to encounter at least one client who has sustained a TBI (Struchen & Clark, 2007).

In medical settings, the role of the social worker is often seen by health care professionals as limited to dealing with patients' social needs such as discharge planning, community referrals, financial arrangements, coordinating family support, advocating for patient's rights, and facilitating support groups (Davies & Connolly, 1995), and addressing the emotional needs of the patients and their families (Craig & Muskat, 2013). Role clarity might be impinged by different factors such as limiting assumption, role blurring, role ambiguity, and hierarchies. For instance, medical social workers' roles might be limited to the assumptions the other members hold with regard to their range of expertise (Jackson & Tangney, 1997). Role clarity is achieved when there is clear information about the expectations and responsibilities of the social work role. Research supports that role clarity is positively correlated with job satisfaction (Lyons, 1971). On the other hand, role ambiguity occurs when there are unclear practice guidelines, poor communication practices, unspecified expectations, and a lack of information regarding how performance is evaluated (Gray & White, 2012).

Medical social workers in interdisciplinary teams might experience role blurring, which occurs when at least two different professionals are qualified to perform similar tasks and these tasks are not delegated to either one of them specifically (Gray & White, 2012). For instance, it has been observed that nurses often assume responsibilities that overlap with social workers' roles in medical settings. Such overlaps include acting as a liaison between the team and the patients' families, discharge planning, making referrals, and providing grief counseling (Burton, 2000; Davies & Connolly, 1995; Hill & Johnson, 1999; Long, Kneafsey, Ryan, & Berry, 2002). This overlap of perceived role responsibilities between nurses and social workers could decrease team efficiency due to the duplication of services for patients and their families (Davis, Milosevic, Baldry, & Walsh, 2004). Previous research has shown that role ambiguity can negatively affect team performance, and can lead to added stress and tension between members (McNeil, Mitchell, & Parker, 2013).

The role of nurses has historically been seen as crucial to the efficient functioning of an interdisciplinary team in a hospital setting. This, in part, has been due to the nature and activities performed by nurses in hospital settings, which "tend to be more related to ... physical care and quality management" of the patient (Holliman, Dziegielewski, & Teare, 2003, p. 230). As such, the roles of nurses are often valued more than those of social workers in interdisciplinary teams in health care settings. Social workers might be susceptible to role ambiguity due in part to the unstructured nature of such teams. This will not only require them to adapt to situations and reprioritize tasks daily, but might also lead to discrepancy between how the social work role is conceptualized by social workers and other team members. Thus, lack of role clarity can significantly lead to heightened workplace stress (House & Rizzo, 1972; Kemery, 2006). On the other hand, when there are clear expectations about roles and responsibilities, workplace stress is reduced (e.g., Emmer, 2003; Mc Auliffe, 2009).

The effectiveness of interdisciplinary teams also depends on collaboration among team members. However, factors such as a clash of professional cultures between team members can prevent effective collaboration (Hall, 2005). Relationships between team members from different disciplines having different knowledge and experience are by their nature unequal. For instance, although primary care physicians acknowledge the importance of addressing patients' psychosocial concerns and needs, they might be hesitant to incorporate social workers because of their perceived lack of time to discuss patients' cases with them (Keefe, Geron, & Enguidanos, 2009). These traditional hierarchies can also affect team members' perceived roles, as they might feel intimidated or less worthy, and thus might be hesitant to speak up about their opinions pertaining to patients' care.

In contrast to the various threats posed to workplace stress and role clarity, perceived respect is an important factor that can contribute to cooperation and effort on behalf of one's team or organization (Boezeman & Ellemers, 2007; Tyler & Blader, 2003). Respect in this context refers to the degree to which the individual is valued as a member of that group. Individuals who feel valued by their group members are more likely to invest in the group and perceive themselves as a contributing member of the group, and are thus more likely to be willing to do more for the group.

Due to the complexity of TBIs, an interdisciplinary approach is seen as the most effective way to deliver treatment and rehabilitation services (Keefe et al., 2009). Although many studies outline potential roles for social workers in such settings (Buck, Sagrati, & Kirzner, 2013; French, Parkinson, &

Massetti, 2011; Moore, 2013), currently there is a lack of research on social workers' perceived role clarity, perceived value of self, and how these might affect their perceived respect and value from members of the interdisciplinary team providing services for TBI and ABI patients and their caregivers.

The aim of this study is to examine the relationships between role clarity, workplace stress, perceived respect, value of self, and team collaboration among social workers working in an interdisciplinary team in a brain injury setting. The hypotheses are as follows:

H1. Role clarity will be negatively associated with workplace stress.

H2. Role clarity will be positively associated with perceived respect, value of self for team, and collaboration.

H3. Team collaboration will be negatively associated with workplace stress.

Method

Sample and procedure

Approval from the University's Human Subject Review Committee was obtained prior to conducting this cross-sectional study. Data were obtained through a convenience sampling method using an anonymous online survey. The survey link was sent electronically to the listserv for the International Network for Social Workers in Acquired Brain Injury (INSWABI) during January 2015, which includes a membership of 120 social workers from various countries. A total of 41 participants responded to the survey (34% response rate). However, 4 respondents were excluded from data analyses because their surveys were less than 30% complete. The total sample included in this study was 37.

As shown in Table 1, the majority of the respondents were female (86.5%), White (86.5%), and between the ages of 25 and 44 (46%). More than one third of the respondents are currently working in hospital rehabilitation (40.5%), primarily with adult patients (86.5%). The majority of respondents (59.5%) have 10 years or more of experience in social work practice in an interdisciplinary brain injury setting. More than half of the respondents (54.1%) have been working in their current employment setting for more than 10 years.

Measures

Dependent variable

In this study, the dependent variable, workplace stress, was measured using the 8-item Workplace Stress Scale (American Institute of Stress, n.d.). This scale was selected for its brevity, succinctness, and applicability to all professions. A sample item is, "I find it difficult to express my opinions or feelings

Table 1. Respondents' characteristics.

Variables	N (37)	%
Gender		
Female	32	86.5
Male	5	13.5
Age range		
25–34	7	18.9
35–44	10	27.0
45–54	7	18.9
55–64	10	27.0
65+	3	8.1
Race/ethnicity		
Caucasian/White/European	32	86.5
Non-White	5	13.5
Current country of employment		
Australia	13	35.1
Canada	8	21.6
Ireland	5	13.5
New Zealand	3	8.1
Sweden	1	2.7
United Kingdom	4	10.8
United States	3	8.1
Number of years working in traumatic brain injury settings		
<1 year	3	8.1
1–5 years	6	16.2
6–10 years	6	16.2
>10 years	22	59.5
Types of current employment setting		
Hospital rehabilitation	15	40.5
Outpatient rehab-hospital based	6	16.2
Outpatient rehab-community based	4	10.8
Community-based	5	13.5
Other	7	18.9
Length of time in current position		
<1 year	3	8.1
1–5 years	7	18.9
6–10 years	7	18.9
>10 years	20	54.1
Types of patient population		
Pediatric	1	2.7
Adults	32	86.5
Both	4	10.8

about my job conditions to my superiors." Items are scored on a 5-point Likert scale ranging from 1 (*never*) to 5 (*very often*). The scores were summed. Scores ranged from 8 to 40, with a low score (<15) indicating low workplace stress, and a high score (>26) indicating severe stress. The Cronbach's alpha in this study is .76.

Independent variables

The independent variables in this study were role clarity, perceived respect, and value of self as a contributing member of the team, along with demographic variables (age, gender, race or ethnicity, current country of employment, number of years working in a brain injury setting, length of employment in current setting, types of employment setting, and types of patient population).

Role clarity was measured with the 6 items from the Rizzo, House, and Lirtzman (1970) questionnaire. This scale was selected for use in this study as it has been shown to yield reliable and valid results in most studies on role perceptions among various work settings across different cultures (e.g., Faucett, Corwyn, & Poling, 2013; Lawrence & Kacmar, 2012; Wu & Norman, 2006). Some wordings were modified in this study. For example, the statement "I feel certain about how much authority I have" from the original questionnaire was modified to "I feel certain about how much authority I have *within the interdisciplinary team*" (the modified words are shown in italics). Items are scored on a 7-point Likert scale ranging from 1 (*strongly disagree*) to 7 (*strongly agree*). Thus, higher scores indicate higher role clarity. The internal reliability of the original scale was .80 (Schuler, Aldag, & Brief, 1977). In this study, the Cronbach's alpha for this scale is .90.

Perceived respect, which refers to the extent to which one feels respected by other professionals within the team, was assessed with an adapted version of the Ellemers, Sleebos, Stam, and de Gilder (2013) Perceived Respect scale. Scale items include "I have a feeling that the professionals in my team respect me for my ways of cooperation." Items are scored on a 5-point Likert scale ranging from 1 (*strongly disagree*) to 5 (*strongly agree*), with higher scores indicating higher perceived respect. In this study Cronbach's alpha for this scale is .80.

Value of self for team was measured with two items adapted by Ellemers et al. (2013) from Heatherton and Polivy's (1991) self-esteem scale. These two items were selected to indicate respondents' perceived value of their contribution to the team's performance. A sample item is "I contribute to the success of my team." Scoring of scale items ranges from 1 (*strongly disagree*) to 5 (*strongly agree*), where higher scores indicate higher value of self as a contributing member for the team. This study reported a Spearman–Brown coefficient alpha of .81.

Interdisciplinary team collaboration was measured using 6 items from the Collaborative Practice Assessment Tool, a valid and reliable tool for assessing levels of interdisciplinary collaboration (Schroder et al., 2011). The original scale was made up of eight subscales that assess various domains pertaining to collaborative practice. For the purpose of this study, items from the Communication and Information Exchange subscale (6 items) were used to assess levels of collaborative practice among team members. Items are scored on a 7-point Likert scale ranging from 1 (*strongly disagree*) to 7 (*strongly agree*). A sample item is "Patients/clients' concerns are addressed effectively through regular team meetings and discussions." Higher scores indicate higher team collaboration. The Cronbach's alpha in this study is .93.

Data analysis

Data were analyzed using SPSS.22. Descriptive statistics for the demographic variables and the independent and dependent variables were generated. The independent and dependent variables were inspected for and met the criterion for normality. Pearson product–moment correlation coefficients were computed to assess the relationships between workplace stress, role clarity, perceived respect, value of self for team, and team collaboration. Multiple regression analysis was conducted to examine which factors contributed to workplace stress and role clarity. Finally, t tests and a one-way analysis of variance (ANOVA) was conducted to examine whether there was any significant difference between the respondents' characteristics with all the primary study variables.

Results

Table 2 shows the means, standard deviations, and correlations for all variables of interest. As indicated in Table 2, there were significant positive correlations between role clarity and perceived respect, value of self as a contributing member of the team, and team collaboration. The positive correlation between role clarity and team collaboration indicates that the more collaboration there is among the team members, the higher their role clarity.

Due to the nonsignificant relationship between workplace stress and the independent variables, regression analysis was not conducted to examine the contributing factors for workplace stress. To further investigate which factors contribute to role clarity, multiple regression analysis was conducted (see Table 3). Due to the relatively small sample size, multiple regression analysis was conducted with only those variables that were significantly associated with role clarity (i.e., perceived respect, value of self for team, and team collaboration). Results showed that the combined factors accounted for 29% of the total variance in role clarity. The most significant predictor variable for

Table 2. Means, standard deviation, and correlation coefficients of variables of interest.

					Correlations		
	M	SD	Role clarity	Perceived respect	Perceived value of self for team	Team collaboration	Length of current employment
Workplace stress	2.40	0.58	−.30	−.28	−.24	−.05	−.05
Role clarity	5.58	1.03	—	.40*	.49**	.43**	.21
Perceived respect	4.13	0.52		—	.33*	.46**	.25
Perceived value of self for team	4.25	0.59			—	.50**	.17
Team collaboration	5.23	1.29				—	.11
Length of current employment							—

*$p < .05$. **$p < .01$.

Table 3. Result of multiple regression analysis predicting role clarity.

Variable	B	t value	p value	R^2	Adjusted R^2	F change
Perceived respect	.198	1.23	.22	.349	.288	5.72**
Value of self for team	.340	2.06	.04*			
Team collaboration	.208	1.19	.24			

*$p < .05$. **$p < .01$.

Table 4. Frequencies of workplace stress by length of employment.

Workplace stress	<5 years	5–10 years	>10 years	Total	%
Very low or fairly low stress	6	4	14	24	64.9
Moderate stress	2	3	5	10	27.0
Severe stress	2	0	1	3	8.1

role clarity was value of self for team, as determined by the standardized coefficient ($\beta = .37$, $t = 2.30$, $p < .05$).

There was no statistically significant difference on the primary study variables by age or gender, length of employment, types of employment settings, or country of employment. The majority of the respondents reported low to fairly low workplace stress (about 65%), and approximately 27% reported a moderate level of stress (as shown in Table 4).

Discussion

The purpose of this study was to investigate the experiences of social workers in an interdisciplinary team in TBI and ABI settings. Overall, the findings of this study showed that factors such as perceived respect from team members, value of self for team, and team collaboration were significantly associated with role clarity. Among these variables, perceived value of self for team emerged as the most significant predictor of role clarity. This suggests that social workers in this study not only have clear expectations about their role in the interdisciplinary team, but perceived themselves as a valued member of the team. This further suggests that the participants generally feel valued and important in their jobs. Additionally, this supports the assumption that an effective interdisciplinary team is one in which members respect each other's expertise and collaborate in the delivery of care. Ellemers et al. (2013) also noted that the degree to which individuals are respected by the team conveys the extent to which the individual is valued as a member of the team and understands his or her potential contribution to the team.

Findings from other studies have also reported that being trusted and respected by other professionals have important implications for the well-being of social workers (Graham & Shier, 2010), and such perceptions can significantly influence an individual's subsequent attitudes and behaviors with respect to their jobs (Legood, McGrath, Searle, & Lee, 2016). Although there was no statistically significant association between role clarity and workplace stress, looking at the correlation coefficients (Table 2) gives a general sense of the direction of the relationship, such that the higher the clarity of role, the lower the workplace stress. It is probable that this lack of association could also be due to the fact that most of the respondents in this study have strong role clarity and low levels of workplace stress as observed in Table 3, or it could be due to the small sample size.

Findings from this study also show that the majority of respondents reported very low or fairly low workplace stress. This might, in part, be due to the role clarity experienced by social workers in the interdisciplinary teams. Previous researchers also report that clarity of role expectations and responsibilities among team members were associated with reduced workplace stress (Emmer, 2003; Mc Auliffe, 2009; McNeil et al., 2013).

As social workers have traditionally collaborated with other disciplines, bringing professional expertise to the psychosocial needs of patients and families, they are uniquely suited to participation in the care of patients with TBI, whose needs are complex and go beyond the provision of medical care. Care provided by members of interdisciplinary teams with diverse skills and experience can also be a very positive experience for the patients or consumers and their families. To reduce workplace stress, there is a need for role clarity among the varied team members. This will also help to reduce duplication between services and improve communication between professionals, which will enable them to provide a more seamless service. Equally important is being valued as a team member who contributes to the success of interdisciplinary efforts. When collaboration works well, it also results in improved services for patients and consumers.

Implications

The findings of this study provide important implications. Due to the complexities of TBI and ABI, which require extensive treatment and rehabilitation services, an interdisciplinary approach can effectively provide treatment and rehabilitation services (Keefe et al., 2009). The social worker is vital to the interdisciplinary process as a core member of the TBI interdisciplinary team. The holistic approaches to health care that also incorporate biopsychosocial, socioecological, and social determinants frameworks to health can be especially beneficial to patients in settings such as those that treat TBI. Training and education of professional social workers should include how to function in interdisciplinary teams.

As each profession has its own culture and sets of values, beliefs, and norms (Hall, 2005), the approach from different perspectives can result in differences among team members with regard to assessment of needs and determining the treatment approach for patients. Respect of each members' expertise and collaborative communication style are vital for the delivery of holistic care for patients in TBI and ABI settings.

Although this study did not find any statistically significant differences in the study variables by country of employment, it is important to note that public perception of a profession might also have an important influence on the vitality and effectiveness of that profession (Reid & Misener, 2001). For instance, if a profession is perceived positively by the public, it will also enhance the credibility of members of that profession among other team members. In countries such as Australia and New Zealand, social work as a profession is publicly recognized and internationally developed (Beddoe & Fraser, 2012). On the other hand, public attitudes toward social work have declined in the United Kingdom, especially after negative reports of social work practices in parts of England, which have undermined public trust further (Laville, 2015). This, in turn, could affect perceptions of the social work role and the competence of social workers in the functioning of inter-disciplinary teams. To counter this, there needs to be active promotion of the profession at both the micro- and macrolevel, such as self-promotion of the profession, as well as endorsement of the social work profession through external sources at the macrolevel.

In medical settings, social workers' roles could sometimes overlap with those of nurses in functions such as making referrals, discharge planning, and providing emotional support to patients and families. Therefore, it is imperative for team members to achieve role clarity with regard to job expectations and responsibilities (Lyons, 1971); the lack of role clarity can lead to workplace stress. Interdisciplinary education supporting holistic care is vital and can benefit members of an interdisciplinary team to improve and sustain collaboration among team members, and help to reduce workplace stress in the interdisciplinary team.

Limitations and conclusion

As with any research, there are certain limitations in this study. Although this is one of the first studies to investigate the role of social workers in interdisciplinary teams that includes an international sample, the small sample size and the convenience sampling method limit the generalizability of the study. Although the study findings report that factors such as perceived respect, team collaboration, and value of self for team increase role clarity, it does not examine whether this leads to job satisfaction. Future research can include factors such as job satisfaction and role overload, and whether these factors are associated with workplace stress. Although the findings suggest that social workers might be more valued and have role clarity in interdisciplinary teams in brain injury settings, future research should compare interdisciplinary teams with other settings such as cancer care, nursing home care, and out-patient clinics, to determine if there are areas of health care where the roles are clearer and the satisfactions are greater.

References

American Institute of Stress. (n.d.). *Workplace stress.* Retrieved from http://www.stress.org/workplace-stress/

Atkinson, L., & Merry, G. (2001). Advances in neurotrauma in Australia 1970–2000. *World Journal of Surgery, 25,* 1224–1229. doi:10.1007/s00268-001-0086-4

Auslander, G. (2001). Social work in health care: What have we achieved? *Journal of Social Work, 1,* 201–222. doi:10.1177/146801730100100206

Barret, G., Sellman, D., & Thomas, J. (2005). *Interprofessional working in health and social care: Professional perspectives.* New York, NY: Palgrave Macmillan.

Beddoe, L. (2011). Health social work: Professional identity and knowledge. *Qualitative Social Work, 12*(1), 24–40. doi:10.1177/1473325011415455

Beddoe, L., & Fraser, H. (2012). Social work in Australasia. In K. H. Lyons, T. Hokenstad, M. Pawar, N. Huegler, & N. Hall (Eds.), *The Sage handbook of international social work* (pp. 421–425). Thousand Oaks, CA: Sage.

Boezeman, E. J., & Ellemers, N. (2007). Volunteering for charity: Pride, respect, and the commitment of volunteer workers. *Journal of Applied Psychology, 92,* 771–781. doi:10.1037/0021-9010.92.3.771

Brain Injury Association of America. (n.d.). Home page. Retrieved from http://www.biausa.org/

Bruner, C. (1991). *Thinking collaboratively: Ten questions and answers to help policy makers improve children's services.* Washington, DC: Education and Human Services Consortium.

Buck, P. W., Sagrati, J. S., & Kirzner, R. S. (2013). Mild traumatic brain injury: A place for social work. *Social Work in Health Care, 52,* 741–751. doi:10.1080/00981389.2013.799111

Burton, C. R. (2000). A description of the nursing role in stroke rehabilitation. *Journal of Advanced Nursing, 32*(1), 174–181. doi:10.1046/j.1365-2648.2000.01411.x

Choi, B. C., & Pak, A. W. (2006). Multidisciplinary, interdisciplinary and transdisciplinary in health research, services, education and policy: 1. Definitions, objectives, and evidence of effectiveness. *Clinical and Investigative Medicine, 29,* 351–364.

Craig, S. L., & Muskat, B. (2013). Bouncers, brokers, and glue: The self-described roles of social workers in urban hospitals. *Health & Social Work, 38*(1), 7–16. doi:10.1093/hsw/hls064

Davies, M., & Connolly, J. (1995). The social worker's role in the hospital: Seen through the eyes of other healthcare professionals. *Health and Social Care in the Community, 3,* 301–309. doi:10.1111/j.1365-2524.1995.tb00031.x

Davis, C., Milosevic, B., Baldry, E., & Walsh, A. (2004). Defining the role of the hospital social worker in Australia: Part 2. A qualitative approach. *International Social Work, 48,* 289–299. doi:10.1177/0020872805051732

Ellemers, N., Sleebos, E., Stam, D., & de Gilder, D. (2013). Feeling included and valued: How perceived respect affects positive team identity and willingness to invest in the team. *British Journal of Management, 24*, 21–37. doi:10.1111/j.1467-8551.2011.00784.x

Emmer, L. (2003). The social worker as part of an interdisciplinary team. *Adolescent Health, 3*(1), 1–3.

Faucett, J., Corwyn, R., & Poling, T. (2013). Clergy role stress: Interactive effects of role ambiguity and role conflict on intrinsic job satisfaction. *Pastoral Psychology, 62*, 291–304. doi:10.1007/s11089-012-0490-8

Feigin, V. L., Theadom, A., Barker-Collo, S., Starkey, N. J., McPherson, K., Michael, K., ... Shanthi, A. (2013). Incidence of traumatic brain injury in New Zealand: A population-based study. *The Lancet Neurology, 12*(1), 53–64. doi:10.1016/s1474-4422(12)70262-4

Fordyce, W. E. (1981). ACRM presidential address on interdisciplinary peers. *Archives of Physical Medicine and Rehabilitation, 62*, 51–53.

French, L. M., Parkinson, G. W., & Massetti, S. (2011). Care coordination in military traumatic brain injury. *Social Work in Health Care, 50*, 501–514. doi:10.1080/00981389.2011.582007

Graham, J. R., & Shier, M. L. (2010). The social work profession and subjective well-being: The impact of a profession on overall subjective well-being. *British Journal of Social Work, 40*, 1553–1572. doi:10.1093/bjsw/bcp049

Gray, F. C., & White, A. (2012). Concept analysis: Case management role confusion. *Nursing Forum, 47*(1), 3–8. doi:10.1111/j.1744-6198.2011.00244.x

Hall, P. (2005). Interprofessional teamwork: Professional cultures as barriers. *Journal of Interprofessional Care, 1*(Suppl.), 188–196. doi:10.1080/13561820500081745

Heatherton, T. F., & Polivy, J. (1991). Development and validation of a scale for measuring state self-esteem. *Journal of Personality and Social Psychology, 60*, 895–910. doi:10.1037/0022-3514.60.6.895

Hill, M. C., & Johnson, J. (1999). An exploratory study of nurses' perceptions of their role in neurological rehabilitation. *Rehabilitation Nursing, 24*, 152–157. doi:10.1002/j.2048-7940.1999.tb02163.x

Holliman, D., Dziegielewski, S., & Teare, R. (2003). Differences and similarities between social work and nurse discharge planners. *Health & Social Workers, 28*, 224–231. doi:10.1093/hsw/28.3.224

House, R., & Rizzo, J. (1972). Role conflict and role ambiguity as critical variables in a model of behavior. *Organizational Behavior and Human Performance, 7*, 467–505. doi:10.1016/0030-5073(72)90030-x

Jackson, A. C., & Tangney, S. (1997). A service mapping approach to the analysis of service use for people with acquired brain injury. *International Perspectives on Social Work in Health Care: Past, Present, and Future, 25*(1–2), 169–192. doi:10.1300/j010v25n01_15

Keefe, B., Geron, S. M., & Enguidanos, S. (2009). Integrating social workers into primary care: Physician and nurse perception of roles, benefits, and challenges. *Social Work in Health Care, 48*, 579–596. doi:10.1080/00981380902765592

Kemery, E. R. (2006). Clergy role stress and satisfaction: Role ambiguity isn't always bad. *Pastoral Psychology, 54*, 561–570. doi:10.1007/s11089-006-0024-3

Keris, V., Lavendelis, E., & Macane, I. (2007). Association between implementation of clinical practice guidelines and outcome for traumatic brain injury. *World Journal of Surgery, 31*, 1352–1355. doi:10.1007/s00268-007-9002

Langois, J. A., Rutland-Brown, W., & Thomas, K. E. (2006). *Traumatic brain injury in the United States, emergency department visits, hospitalizations, and deaths.* Atlanta, GA: Centers for Disease Control and Prevention, National Center for Injury Prevention and Control.

Laville, S. (2015, March 3) Professionals blamed Oxfordshire girls for their sexual abuse, report finds. *The Guardian*. Retrieved from www.theguardian.com/society/2015/mar/03/professionals-blamed-oxfordshire-girls-for-their-sexual-abuse-report-finds

Lawrence, E., & Kacmar, K. M. (2012). Leader-member exchange and stress: The mediating role of job involvement and role conflict. *Journal of Behavioral & Applied Management, 14*(1), 39–52.

Legood, A., McGrath, M., Searle, R., & Lee, A. (2016). Exploring how social workers experience and cope with public perception of their profession. *British Journal of Social Work*. Advance online publicaton. doi:10.1093/bjsw/bcv139

Long, A. F., Kneafsey, R., Ryan, J., & Berry, J. (2002). The role of the nurse within the multi-professional rehabilitation team. *Journal of Advanced Nursing, 37*(1), 70–78. doi:10.1046/j.1365-2648.2002.02059.x

Lyons, T. F. (1971). Role clarity, need for clarity, satisfaction, tension, and withdrawal. *Organizational Behavior and Human Performance, 6*, 99–110. doi:10.1016/0030-5073(71)90007-9

Mc Auliffe, C. (2009). Experiences of social workers within an interdisciplinary team in the intellectual disability sector. *Critical Social Thinking: Policy and Practice, 1*, 125–143.

McNeil, K. A., Mitchell, R. J., & Parker, V. (2013). Interprofessional practice and professional identity threat. *Health Sociology Review, 22*, 291–307. doi:10.5172/hesr.2013.22.3.291

Menon, D. K., Schwab, K., Wright, D. W., & Maas, A. I. (2010). Position statement: Definition of traumatic brain injury. *Archives of Physical Medicine and Rehabilitation, 91*, 1637–1640. doi:10.1016/j.apmr.2010.05.017

Moore, M. (2013). Mild traumatic brain injury: Implications for social work research and practice with civilian and military populations. *Social Work in Health Care, 52*, 498–518. doi:10.1080/00981389.2012.714447

Morris, S., Ridley, S., Lecky, F. E., Munro, V., & Christensen, M. (2008). Determinants of hospital costs associated with traumatic brain injury in England and Wales. *Anaesthesia, 63*, 499–508. doi:10.1111/j.1365-2044.2007.05432.x

Orchard, C. A., Curran, V., & Kabene, S. (2005). Creating a culture for interdisciplinary collaborative professional practice. *Medical Education Online, 10*, 10–11. doi:10.3402/meo.v10i0.4387

Prigatano, G. P. (1999). *Principles of neuropsychological rehabilitation*. New York, NY: Oxford University Press.

Reid, W. J., & Misener, E. (2001). Social work in the press: A cross-national study. *International Journal of Social Welfare, 10*, 194–201. doi:10.1111/1468-2397.00172

Rizzo, J. R., House, R. J., & Lirtzman, S. I. (1970). Role conflict and ambiguity in complex organizations. *Administrative Science Quarterly, 15*, 150–163. doi:10.2307/2391486

Roozenbeek, B., Maas, A., & Menon, D. K. (2013). Changing patterns in the epidemiology of traumatic brain injury. *Nature Reviews Neurology, 9*, 231–236. doi:10.1038/nrneurol.2013.22

Russell, W. R., & Smith, A. (1961). Post-traumatic amnesia in closed head injury. *Archives of Neurology, 5*(1), 4–17. doi:10.1001/archneur.1961.00450130006002

Sander, A. M., & Constantinidou, F. (2008). The interdisciplinary team. *Journal of Head Trauma Rehabilitation, 23*, 271–272. doi:10.1097/01.htr.0000336839.68585.0f

Schroder, C., Medves, J., Paterson, M., Byrnes, V., Chapman, C., O'Riordan, A., … Kelly, C. (2011). Development and pilot testing of the collaborative practice assessment tool. *Journal of Interprofessional Care, 25*, 189–195. doi:10.3109/13561820.2010.532620

Schuler, R. S., Aldag, R. J., & Brief, A. P. (1977). Role conflict and ambiguity: A scale analysis. *Organizational Behavior and Human Performance, 20*, 111–128. doi:10.1016/0030-5073(77)90047-2

Smith, D. H., Hicks, R. R., Johnson, V. E., Bergstrom, D. A., Cummings, D. A., Noble, L. J., … Edward, D. C. (2015). Pre-clinical traumatic brain injury common data elements: Toward a common language across laboratories. *Journal of Neurotrauma, 32,* 1725–1735. doi:10.1089/neu.2014.3861

Strasser, D. C., Uomoto, J. M., & Smits, S. J. (2008). The interdisciplinary team and polytrauma rehabilitation: Prescription for partnership. *Archives of Physical Medicine and Rehabilitation, 89,* 179–181. doi:10.1016/j.apmr.2007.06.774

Struchen, M. A., & Clark, A. N. (2007). *Systematic approach to social work practice: Working with clients with traumatic brain injury.* Houston, TX: Baylor College of Medicine.

Supiano, K. P., & Berry, P. H. (2013). Developing interdisciplinary skills and professional confidence in palliative care social work students. *Journal of Social Work Education, 49,* 387–396.

Tyler, T. R., & Blader, S. L. (2003). The group engagement model: Procedural justice, social identity, and cooperative behavior. *Personality & Social Psychology Review, 7,* 349–361. doi:10.1207/s15327957pspr0704_07

Wu, L., & Norman, I. (2006). An investigation of job satisfaction, organizational commitment and role conflict and ambiguity in a sample of Chinese undergraduate nursing students. *Nurse Education Today, 26,* 304–314. doi:10.1016/j.nedt.2005.10.011

Index

9 780367 892142